Qigong
for
healing and relaxation

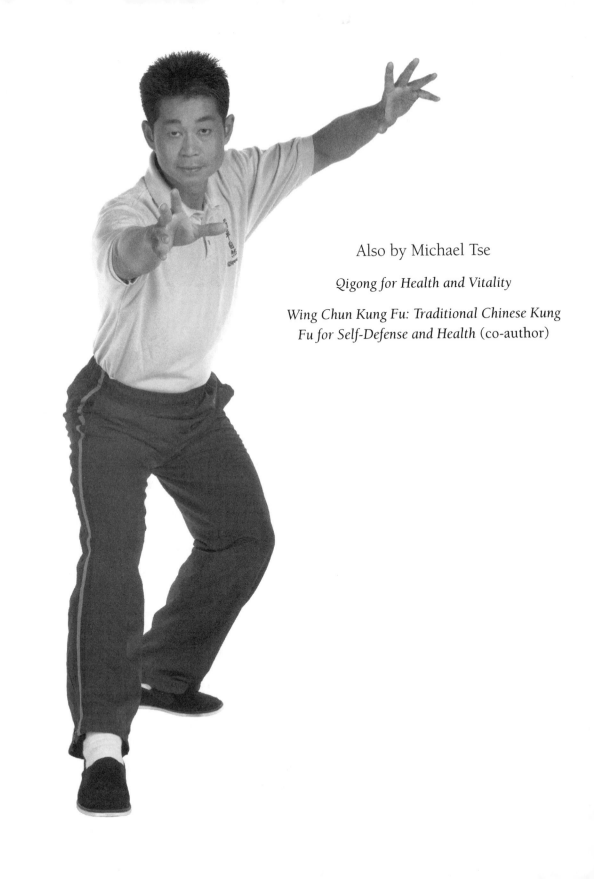

Also by Michael Tse

Qigong for Health and Vitality

Wing Chun Kung Fu: Traditional Chinese Kung Fu for Self-Defense and Health (co-author)

Qigong *for* healing and relaxation:

Simple Techniques for Feeling Stronger, Healthier, and More Relaxed

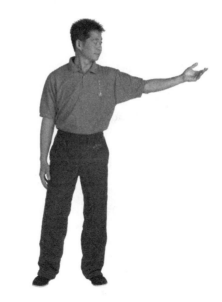

Michael Tse

St. Martin's Griffin ✖ New York

613.7/98

Library of Congress Cataloging-in-Publication Data Available Upon Request

ISBN 0-312-34026-5
EAN 978-0-312-34026-1

Edited by Barbara Kiser
Page design and make up by Paul Saunders
Photographs by Jon Stewart
Illustrations by Rodney Paull

First published in the United Kingdom by Piatkus

First U.S. Edition: February 2005

10 9 8 7 6 5 4 3 2 1

About the author

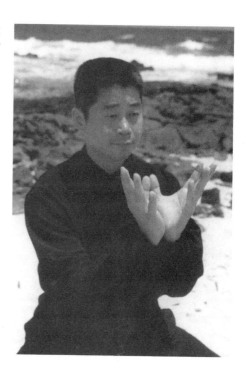

HONG KONG-BORN Michael Tse has studied Qigong and martial arts for over 30 years with some of the world's most renowned masters. His Qigong Sifu (teacher), Grandmaster Yang Meijun, passed away in China in 2002 at the age of 104.

She taught him not only most of the surviving forms from the 1,800-year-old Kunlun Dayan (Wild Goose) system of Qigong, but also passed on the Qigong healing skills for which she was so famous.

With this knowledge of Qigong, and his study of Chinese philosophy, history and martial arts, Tse created a series of Qigong exercises called Healthy Living Gong in 1996. This book covers the first part of these imaginative and highly effective Qigong healing tools.

Michael Tse founded the Tse Qigong Centre in England in 1990 along with the popular *Qi Magazine*, which gives Western readers a deeper insight and understanding of Chinese culture. He divides his time between Hawaii, where he founded a centre in 2001, and England. He also gives seminars around the world, helping to promote the Qigong skills that have enriched his own life so deeply and have proven a successful way to health and happiness for so many others.

IN THE PAST, people did not have access to paper and pen like we do today. China's earliest writing was done on slips of bamboo that were then stitched together to become a 'book'. You can imagine how heavy some of them must have been. So when learning movements in martial arts and Qigong, people would create a poem to remember the meaning of the movements. Below is a poem created by one of my Qigong students and it catches the essence of the form of Qigong in this book. If you can learn this poem by heart, then it can help you understand how to do each movement and also its benefit.

Poetry in Motion

Collect the Qi
From left and right
To Dantian, sway
From side to side.

Sweep hands to both sides
And stand very proud
To separate the fog
And look for a cloud.

Let's search for fish
By the side of the lake
Keep head above waist
To get rid of headaches.

When golden dragon
Stretches its claws
Move waist and arms
Without pause.

Old tree winds its roots
To sink your Qi
Imagine how strong
Your legs will soon be.

Jade ladder climbs
Into the sky;
It helps when your blood pressure
Is too high.

Of a beautiful ball
Keep a gentle hold
To rid yourself of bronchitis and cold.

When you look for treasure
At the bottom of the chest
It's not the money but good health
In which you invest.

Swing the child left and right
Shift weight and bend knees
It gets rid of tennis elbow
And circulates your Qi.

VERA EXTERNEST
Qigong Student, 2003

Acknowledgements

I WOULD LIKE TO give special thanks to my wife Jessica and my son Anthony, who both stimulate my thinking and make me laugh. I would like to thank my teachers, Yang Meijun, Ip Chun, Wu Chun Yuen and Chen Xiao Wang for their knowledge and their dedication to their skill. I thank my father, Tse Bing Kei, who passed away in February 2003, and who helped me understand loyalty, wisdom, hard work and family feeling. And I would also like to thank the rest of my family, including my mother, sister and all my brothers.

Thanks also to those people helping in the Tse Qigong Centre, including Darryl Moy, Martin Gale, Sarah Moy and Caroline Garvey. Their loyalty is never in doubt. I would like to thank all the instructors who take care of and assist in my classes while I travel, helping to pass on the Healthy Living Gong skill to others: John Hayes, Julian Wilde, Glenn Gossling, Martin Rooney, Sharhiar Sepangi, Chi Man Tang, Mike Baker, Peter Walfisz, Simon Bedford, Khim Chang, Kate Britton and Dana Walfisz. There are many, many more, both instructors and students around the world, whom I would also like to thank – their names too numerous to list here. I know they always support me and I am proud to watch them grow and their students grow.

Thanks also to Jennie Cunningham, Adam Wallace, Steve Casano, Kahi Wight and Brandon Eugenio, Khim Guan, Barbara Bigsby, and

Olga Gonzalez for their proofreading and comments. Lastly, I would also like to thank everyone at Piatkus Books for offering me this opportunity to share more knowledge with all of you, particularly Judy Piatkus, Gill Bailey, Jane Burton, Anna Crago and Isabelle Almeida. Without all of your support, I could not have finished this book.

Contents

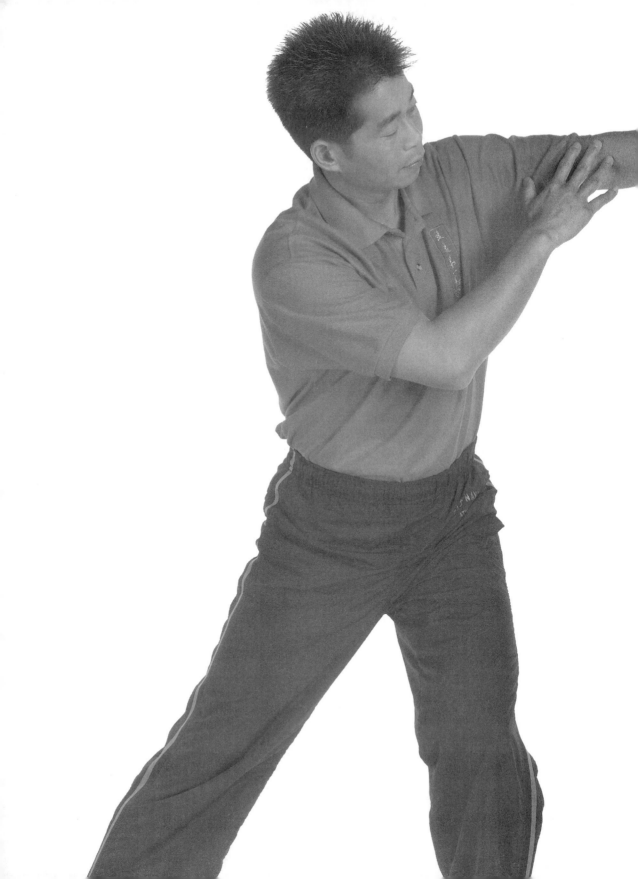

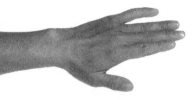

Introduction

QIGONG ARE TRADITIONAL Chinese healing exercises that harnesses Qi – vital energy, or the life force – through breathing techniques, movements, postures and meditation. Practising Qigong helps you to balance passive and active forces (Yin and Yang), allowing Qi to flow freely and harmoniously. If you are a complete newcomer to Qigong, you'll find a full explanation of it in Chapter 1.

Healthy Living Gong is a set of Qigong exercises that I began to develop in 1996, based upon over 30 years of my Qigong Taijiquan, Wing Chun and Northern Shaolin (Chun Yuen) experience as well as knowledge gained from healing people through Qigong therapy, Chinese philosophy, Yijing (*Book of Changes*) and Chinese medicine theory.

There are three parts to the Healthy Living Gong exercises. Each set has nine single movements and one walking exercise, which is a variation on one of the standing movements. Although called 'standing movements', actually they involve moving your waist, moving your body backwards, forwards and up and down. The walking movement is for developing coordination and orientation and creating more energy. Each movement is individual and should be repeated a number of times – in contrast to forms where you do each movement once in a series.

I began to develop Healthy Living Gong because I had been aware for some time that most people beginning Qigong were unable to learn the more complicated forms that I taught, like Wild Goose Qigong or Jade

Pillar Gong, especially if they were ill or did not have much experience in movement. I saw the opportunity to introduce some of the movements from the first set of Healthy Living Gong at a workshop I was teaching in London in late 1996.

My students and I had just given a demonstration of skills they had learned, but these were all quite advanced Qigong forms. I began, with the workshop participants, the first six movements I had created, called *Collecting Qi to the Dantian, Separating the Fog to Look for the Clouds, Catching Fish by the Side of the Lake, Golden Dragon Stretches Its Claws, Old Tree with Winding Roots* and *Jade Ladder Climbing to the Sky*.

I found that the people liked the movements very much, and they picked them up easily. As each movement was individual and was for helping a particular part of the body or health problem, they could concentrate on whichever movement was the most relevant for them.

Today, I regularly use the Healthy Living Gong exercises in my Qigong healing practise, rather than showing my patients a Qigong form to do. This is because a single movement will focus on a particular health problem more deeply than doing a Qigong form. A Qigong form is more about making the Qi smooth in the body. For instance, if someone has a back problem, I will show them *Looking for Treasure at the Bottom of the Chest*, as this movement works with the kidneys, back and waist. For someone who has breathing problems or asthma, I will maybe show them *Holding the Beautiful Ball* or *Separating the Fog to Look for the Clouds*, as both of these exercises work for the lungs and posture.

I have now developed three sets of Healthy Living Gong exercises. This book concentrates on the first set, which will help you to develop your health and open your body's healing potential. In this set we are working for relaxation and balance. The second set is all about coordination and fitness and includes lots of waist and leg movements. The third is for encouraging strength and power, with some movements actually based upon martial art movements, although done with a Qigong attitude and an emphasis on health.

Among the inspirations for Healthy Living Gong are my observations of nature and stories within Chinese culture, like fables or some event in history. People say that when they practise these exercises, they can actually visualise what the movement should be like based upon the names. All the exercises in the book are shown in detailed photo sequences with descriptions.

When you first learn the movements, you should try to practise them in order. That will help you to cover all aspects of movement, breathing and relaxation. Later, once you are familiar with them all, you can choose the exercises that are most suitable for your condition. An index of benefits of each exercise is shown with its coordinating movement in Appendix I.

For each movement there is an explanation of its benefit to the body, its history and the area of concentration. This will help you to understand what you need to focus on and how the movement will help heal the body. Qigong helps us to heal ourselves through movement, breathing and relaxation. In order to be healthy, we need to move. The human body is made to move, otherwise we would not have joints and muscles and a skeleton. However, we need to move in a relaxed way. If we are not relaxed, tension will block the Qi from moving in the body. If the Qi cannot move, the problem will just stay and will get worse and worse, like a traffic jam that is not cleared from the road.

If we don't move, we will not be healthy – even if we take all kinds of vitamins and herbs. Many people think only of the external body. They try to be slimmer, have good muscles, even have plastic surgery to look better. They do not realise, though, that the condition of the internal body (the organs, Qi and blood) is reflected in the condition of the external body.

For instance, if the kidneys are not healthy, the hair will be dry and will fall out easily. If there is a problem with the lungs, the skin will be dry and in poor condition. If the liver is weak, a person will feel cold and their hands will be thin and have a yellow colour and they will start to have problems with their eyesight. If the heart is unhealthy, a person can have acne, or feel dizzy or faint. If there is a problem in the spleen, the lips will lack colour, be white, chapped and dry. So no matter how much make-up you wear or weight training you do, eventually you will not be able to hide the problem. It will come out in other ways. (See Chapter 8, 'How Palms and Face Relate to Health', for further information on this.)

Qigong helps to make us healthy from the inside out. This is because Qigong movement helps to release negative Qi in the body and gather fresh Qi. It helps to open the channels in the body and stimulate the circulation. Blood carries Qi, so if we do not move, the blood will not flow well and Qi will be stagnant. When Qi does not flow, this is how illness develops in the body. It is like taking a bath in the same bathwater every day for a year. Will you get clean? Of course not!

Our bodies are the same. We need to change the energy and clean our internal body in order for it to be healthy. When the inside is healthy, the outside will show this. For myself, no matter what kind of illness or injury I have, I will always choose Qigong to heal myself.

If you have a deeper understanding of how Qigong works to make you healthy, then you will be able to move more accurately within each exercise and develop your skill more quickly. Many people today think that they are healthy, but this is not necessarily good health from a Qigong point of view. I discuss good and bad health in more detail in Chapter 2 and also introduce more about the history and philosophy of Qigong in Chapter 3.

Healthy Living Gong is for anyone. The exercises cover all different aspects of movement – slow and fast, easy and difficult. Healthy Living Gong works on helping different problems, including insomnia, high or low blood pressure, back problems, arthritis, stress and worry, by moving specific parts of the body in a special way. It will also help you relax and be more calm. Of course, these exercises are not only for people who have problems with their health; they are also for anyone who wants to maintain good health and for healers wanting to make their Qi level stronger.

People who heal others give away a lot of their energy, so it is easy to feel tired and even ill if you do not release the sick energy you take on from the patient you are healing. If you practise Healthy Living Gong daily, you will improve your health and have a lot of energy. The most important thing for healing others is to be healthy yourself. Otherwise you will pass on the ill energy instead of healthy energy to your patients.

Grandmaster Yang Meijun, my Sifu or teacher, taught me this. She lived to be 104 and every day she practised her Qigong skills to keep her healthy and flexible. She was known throughout China for her skill in healing. However, even though she began practising Wild Goose Qigong when she was 13, she did not begin to heal others until she was over 70 years old. By this time her Qi had become very strong and her understanding of the body, philosophy and how Qi works was exceptional. Not many people today can get to this level. You can read more about this in Chapter 9.

I learned not only Qigong from my Sifu, but also my healing skill. She taught me that you cannot only do soft Qigong movements; you also need more active or difficult movements to balance the soft ones. This is the essence of Yin and Yang. If we only do Yin things, the body will be too weak. If we only practise Yang movement, the body will have too much fire or excitement and will not calm down. (See Chapter 4 for more information on Yin and Yang.) The Qigong she taught me is the Kunlun Dayan Qigong system, which dates from the Jin Dynasty over 1,800 years ago. It covers many forms, including some long, some short, some soft, some hard. I mention some of these throughout the book, like *Green Sea Swimming Dragon Gong* and *Wild Goose Qigong*. The system also covers many different kinds of meditation and healing skills.

It is because of my many years' practise and understanding of the Kunlun Dayan (Wild Goose) Qigong system that I could create Healthy Living Gong. Healthy Living Gong is based upon the principles of the Kunlun Dayan Qigong system in that we use movement for healing, not visualisation. We do not have to think or try to direct the Qi because the movements carry the Qi to where we want it to go. That is why the Chinese government promoted Dayan Qigong as one of the top ten 'healthy' Qigong styles.

Another principle is that we focus directly on the internal organs by bringing Qi to the channels and acupuncture points through movement. So it also covers some knowledge of Traditional Chinese Medicine theory.

For Qigong to heal the body, the most important thing is to be relaxed so that Qi can flow and the mind can calm down. Today we all have a lot of stress and tension in our lives. The longer we carry this tension with us, the more health problems we may have. However, when you do the first movement, *Collecting Qi to the Dantian*, you find all the tension going from your body. Relaxation is important for beginners and

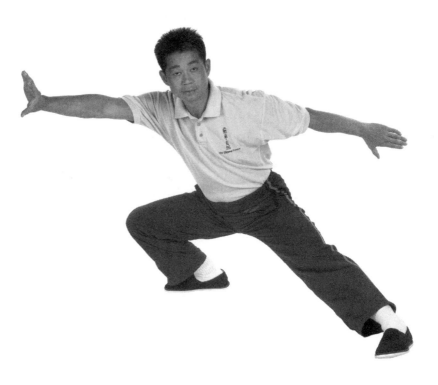

advanced practitioners alike. Breathing and meditation are also crucial for good health (see Chapters 7 and 12).

Healthy Living Gong is good for beginners who have never done any kind of Qigong movement before, but it will also benefit those practised in the discipline, as it will help develop the Qi more strongly in the body. It will bring you to a more advanced Qigong level, allowing you to understand how to heal illnesses. If we can learn how to heal ourselves, we do not need to worry about health problems.

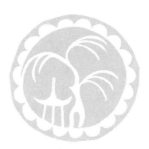

What is Qigong?

THESE DAYS, MANY people already know something about Qigong, so I find I don't have to explain it every time I mention it. But when I first moved from Hong Kong to England in 1988 to teach, things were very different. Most Britons only knew about Tai Chi (Taijiquan), and they thought that it was the same thing as Qigong. Qigong is now popular around the world, and there are many different ideas of what it is. Whatever your concept of Qigong, I would like to give you the right definition.

Qigong is an ancient Chinese practice that works to make us healthier. *Qi* (pronounced 'chee') means vital energy; *Gong* means work. So Qigong is an exercise that works on our vital energy. Vital energy is our life force and without it we cannot survive. Qigong is a way to make us healthier and allow us to live longer by creating extra Qi in the body to make the Qi we were born with stronger. Qigong is also a way of guiding our own healing and bringing our body back into harmony with nature.

There are many countries and cultures that have their own ways of working with Qi or vital energy. However, what makes Qigong different from others is that it is based on the principles of Traditional Chinese Medicine (TCM), which is, in turn, based upon the understanding of the Yin/Yang and Five Element theory, acupuncture points, meridians and the Dantian (the centre of our body, where Qi stored). This knowledge is only found in TCM and in Chinese martial arts. This is why Qigong is a Chinese skill.

Many ways, one way

There many different styles of Qigong, originating from five schools of thought: Daoism, Buddhism, Confucianism, martial and medical (healing). However, all have the same principle of making the vital energy stronger and the body healthy.

Qigong dates back over 3,000 years. During this time, ancient Chinese people lived along the Yellow River, and they had to find ways to survive in that area. As there was a lot of water there and often flooding, the climate was very damp. The people suffered a lot of problems with their joints, like arthritis and rheumatism, because the damp got inside their bodies. It is the same today in many colder countries, such as Britain, Canada, Russia and the north of China. When the damp gets inside the body, it tends to stay in the joints, just like the dust in your house collects in the corners where it is difficult to clean.

These ancient people had to find a way to live in their damp environment, but what could they do? They found the best way was the same as cleaning the dust from our clothes or rugs: to shake them clean. But how do we shake the body? It is easy. All we have to do is move. The ancient Chinese created many different kinds of movements, some of which were like a dance and others which were based upon observations from nature and movements from animals.

These movements might have started in the same way as, Polynesians, Africans and Australian Aborigines created their own cultural dances. However, whereas these cultures danced to commune with nature or tell a story, the movements that these peoples created were particularly for health. These peoples had their own ways to move the body to create internal heat in order to clear dampness and illnesses. This has been documented through old drawings found on bronze vessels and silk (see opposite, above).

Qigong is good for more than getting rid of damp in the joints, however. It helps to balance the body and alleviates all kinds of conditions such as stomach ache, poor circulation, backache, headaches and so on. It releases negative energy and stiffness, so when the ancient Chinese people moved in this special way, they felt lighter and happier and had more energy.

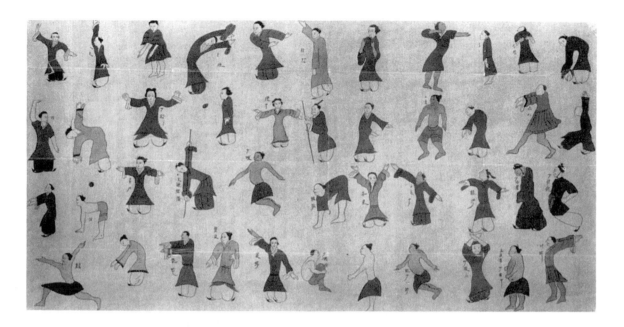

As time went by, the movements and dances began to evolve into a more systemised skill. The people of the Yellow River were great observers of nature. So they came to understand that there are two sides to everything. They saw that as summer passes, winter comes; breathing in, we must then breathe out; we have life, but we also have death. They called this phenomenon Yin and Yang, or the observation of opposites. Yin means dark, soft, hidden, slow, and represents the female. Yang means bright, hard, open, fast, and represents the male. The concept that everything in nature has an opposing force is the foundation of all Chinese culture. It is also the basis of all developments in Chinese medicine, cooking, Qigong, martial arts and philosophy.

Around the same time that Qigong began, these concepts were compiled in a book called the *Yijing*. *Yi* means change and *Jing* means classic book, so the title means *The Classic of Change*. (You may know the book as the *I Ching* or *Book of Changes*.) The *Yijing* is about everything in the universe and how things change, and how this change is based upon the principle of Yin and Yang.

A western Han painting showing the earliest form of Qigong, Daoyin.

Movement and stillness

Following this principle, if we accept that movement is good for the body, we can accept that stillness is also good for the body. Therefore, if we want to be healthy, we must know how to move and also how to be still. Qigong is Yang, as it is moving. Meditation is Yin, as it is still.

Meditation is a resting for the body and mind. When we get tired, we need to rest or sleep. Resting can recharge energy, but in ancient times, people found that the best way to rest was to be somewhere between consciousness and unconsciousness – neither too awake nor too sleepy. Closing the eyes helps the body and mind relax better and helps to exclude outside stimulations and let the mind be at rest and empty.

For many people, though, this was difficult. So different methods to help people forget the active mind and to focus their energy began to develop. Some of these included concentrating on breathing or the Dantian (the place in our body where Qi is stored), or mentally chanting a special phrase or poem, all aimed to empty the mind so that a person could become one with nature. (See Chapter 12 for further information.)

When a person is in tune and balanced with nature, it means nature can recharge your energy and help to restore harmony to the body and mind. When the mind is calm, it is very good for the health. With a calm mind, you will become very clear about everything around you and you will see not just what is in front of you, but will know your direction for the future. Meditation can help you to become a wise person.

When the ancient Chinese people practised both movement and meditation, they found that there was something moving inside their bodies which made them feel good and strong. This was Qi. The more they practised, the stronger and healthier they became. So Qigong began to include meditation as well as movement.

Movement released the negative energy from the body, gathered fresh new Qi from nature and opened the channels for this fresh Qi to circulate. Meditation was for storing the newly gathered Qi so that it could be used later as the body needed it. Therefore, working with Qi is Qigong, but the main aim for doing Qigong is to be healthy. Movement without gathering and storing Qi is not Qigong, because this just releases Qi.

When people run or do aerobics or fitness training, they are using energy and releasing negative energy. But this kind of exercising does not help them recover and replace sick Qi with fresh, healthy Qi. Releasing negative energy is vital to good health, but you also have to gather and store new Qi. This is what makes us healthy, and this is what makes Qigong special.

Qigong can help you live longer by making you healthier. If you are ill, it can give you strength to fight the problem, just as a friend can help you when you are in trouble it can help make you well, so you can have a better and happier life. Meditation will calm your mind and make you relaxed. It will allow the Qi to settle and be stored in the Dantian so that you will be stronger and have more positive energy.

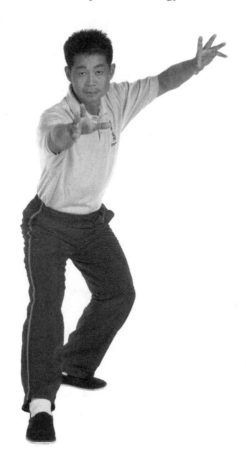

2 Good Health, Bad Health

W HAT DOES BEING healthy mean? Many people will say they are healthy, or will modify it a bit to say – 'I am very healthy, apart from my heart.' I once asked a Western-trained health expert this question. The answer he gave me was very long and full of complicated medical terms. Ordinary people would not be able to grasp what he meant.

Luckily, I think we ourselves can find out the answer to the question of what it means to be healthy. For me, if someone has a clear mind, sleeps properly, eats what they like, functions well physically and has enough energy to do the things they need to do, their health is OK. This is quite true: as long as you are mentally and physically capable and can do what you want, then you are healthy.

For instance, if you have to climb up a ladder to fix something and find that you feel dizzy when you go up, it means your blood circulation is low and so you are not healthy. If you bend forwards or backwards and find your back is stiff or hurts, then you have a problem. Of course, it can just be a small problem and easily fixed by just moving about a little. But if we are not careful, small problems can become big problems.

In the first stages of a physical problem, we tend to stiffen up. Pain usually comes later on and is a sign that there is something physically wrong. We can also suffer from mental problems. For example, if someone tells you something very simple, such as to meet them at a certain time, the majority of people will be able to remember this straight away or will write it in their diary to make sure they remember. Other people might forget straight away. Of course, they might have been doing something else and not paying attention. However, if they did pay attention and still forgot, then this kind of forgetfulness indicates a lack in brain function. This is because there is not enough Qi to nourish the brain, which is reliant on the health and good function of the kidneys to feed it. This is also one reason that people lose their short-term memory as they age, and only remember what has happened in the past. It is because they do not have enough Qi to feed both their mind and body.

If your mental energy is not strong enough, then you may find you cannot concentrate on things like reading a book or newspaper. If you find you cannot understand when someone is talking to you, but other people can understand that person easily, then you have a listening problem. However, it is not a listening problem in that you cannot hear the sound itself. It is because the messages are not passing through to your brain. This means that your Qi is weak. So you need to practise Qigong to gather healthy Qi and to practise meditation to calm your mind and bring more Qi to your brain. This will then develop your mental energy.

To be healthy, you also need to be physically fit and strong so you can essentially do whatever you want to do. Sometimes, when your energy is low, you might not be able to do certain things that you can do normally. For example, when your energy levels are high, you might be able to stand on one leg without any problem. Yet on another day, you might not be able to do it at all. To become healthier, you have to work on the movements you have difficulty with, as it shows that there is a weakness in the body.

This is a point on which Chinese and Western thinking differ. Chinese believe that if there is a problem, like a stiff shoulder or back, we should move more to heal it. When we move, we increase the circulation and allow more Qi to come in to help alleviate the problem. However, Western medicine may tell you not to move at all or to wear a support. People will often tell me that their doctor said they should not move the part of the body that they are having problems with. Some even tell me that their doctor has urged them to have surgery to 'fix' the muscle or painful joint. I have had many people come to me after surgery to ask for help as their problem became even worse. This kind of radical intervention will often make the problem worse, as it means that little or no Qi will go to that area for healing. Even if a joint is locked, we should try to move as much as we can. This means Qi will still go to that area to help heal the problem. The more Qi, the more we can move. The more we move, the more Qi can go there. Whereas, if we cut the joints and tendons, this also cuts the channels which are roadways for Qi and blood. This then makes healing much more difficult and can mean even more stiffness and pain.

Your body is like a car. All the lights on the dashboard have a function and should work. When some of the lights do not work, you should fix them, otherwise they might affect the running of the car. But whereas you can trade in a car any time there is a problem, you only have one body; and despite advances in science, you cannot yet trade it in. Perhaps you can change some parts of it, but it will not be as good as the original.

Good Qi, sick Qi

Good Qi is essential for good health. It makes you feel more energetic, stronger and healthier. But while good Qi is good for the body, there is also sick Qi, and this – following the principle of Yin and Yang – must be bad for the body. The Chinese name for sick Qi is *Bing Qi*, and the name for good Qi is *Hao Qi*.

Good Qi is fresh air. Fresh air gives us energy and comes from nature. When you go on holiday to a beautiful beach or the countryside or the mountains, you will feel good and it will lift your spirit. This is because there is plenty of fresh air.

You can also find energy from sunshine, animals and people, music, food and certain fragrances, for instance. These last things, however, tend to stimulate your energy rather than give you more Qi. Therefore, the major way to get good Qi is still from fresh air. We depend on it for survival, after all. You can listen to good music, which makes you feel good, but you cannot listen to it without air, as you will not be able to live. Food will give you energy, but you also need energy to break it down and digest it and convert it to useful Qi. You can have lots of sunshine, but without fresh air it is useless to you.

So fresh air is the most vital part of Qi. Think of a Chinese stir-fry dish. We think of a combination of chicken and green vegetables as a chicken dish, but without the chicken it is no longer a chicken dish. Even if you use a lot of soy sauce, spring onions and garlic, it will still not be a chicken dish. Some ingredients are the main element and some are just extra. So, even though you can still obtain Qi from other sources, fresh air is the most important ingredient.

For high-quality Qi, it is very important that the air you breathe is fresh. If you breathe air that comes through a ventilation system, you can still get Qi, but the quality is not as good as fresh air from nature. Sometimes you see old people live longer, even without practising Qigong or any other exercises, if the area where they live has plenty of good, fresh air. The better the air, the more Qi it contains.

And through Qigong, you can gather more fresh Qi into your body.

It is like trying to collect water from the tap. How much you get depends on whether you use a big bucket or a small cup. It also depends on the condition of the bucket or cup you use.

When sick Qi comes into your body, it will make you feel uncomfortable or even ill. It could be polluted air from car fumes, rotten waste or a refuse tip, or somewhere with poor ventilation, too much heat, sick animals or sick people. You should avoid these whenever possible. For example, when you are walking down the street, you may suddenly notice a strange smell that makes you feel sick. This is sick or negative Qi, so you should move away and keep your distance from it to avoid taking it in.

Once I went to an antique warehouse in Xian, China. It was very old and dusty and even though it was mostly in the open air, with just a covered roof, I began to feel damp inside and not so well. I knew this was not a healthy place to be in, and so I decided to leave. When I went back to my hotel room, I felt tired and had a headache. The next day I was ill and had a fever and the flu from which it took a few days for me to completely recover. Old, damp and dusty places can create a lot of sick Qi.

Sometimes you might bump into somebody whom you would rather avoid, but there is no way around the situation. Maybe you work in a hospital or are in an office where a lot of people smoke and are not very healthy. Of course, in this kind of situation, you can't really avoid contact with people who are ill. And maybe you notice after seeing them that you feel as if all your energy is gone and you feel tired and weak. This is because the other person's energy is not healthy and also because some of their emotion has been released to you.

Have you ever been in a situation where someone is talking to you and telling you about their problems? If you are more healthy than them, then you will take on all their negative energy and will not feel well afterwards. At the same time, your good Qi will have passed to them, and they will feel better. In this kind of situation, the only thing you can do is practise Qigong to gather more fresh energy and to release the sick energy you have taken in.

People and animals are the same. If they are not well and you come into contact with them, you may be ill later on. If you are strong and healthy you might be able to withstand this, but you will still lose some Qi. The best thing to do is listen to your body. When you do not feel well, go out to practise your Qigong and then you will definitely feel better. Gathering good Qi means being able to take fresh Qi from the environment. If you can practise in a place that has some trees and grass or water, then it will help you gather more Qi and be healthy. Certain environments offer more Qi than others. A lake or a forest will have more Qi than a city park, but the park will offer more Qi than a room in a building.

Sometimes, though, we cannot always go outside to practise, or to start with some people will feel shy. However, if we always practise inside with the windows closed, the benefit we get from Qigong will be much less. If you do practise inside, then open a window to let in fresh air. Still you should try to practise outside more as it will be much easier to gather fresh Qi from nature. Only by gathering fresh Qi and replacing the sick Qi in our bodies can we maintain our health.

Philosophy of Qigong

W E PRACTISE QIGONG for good health, but what is the philosophy behind it all? Essentially, it is to live your life so you stay calm, peaceful and are in harmony with nature. This is based upon the thinking of Daoism, Confucianism (Ru Jia) and Buddhism.

If someone practises their Qigong forms and meditation every day, they will attain good health. However, if something traumatic happens in their life, for example they lose their job, a relative dies or they have financial difficulties, they may lose their balance and heart. After this, they may become ill or depressed; and then they may ask themselves, 'How can I be ill, when I am still practising Qigong every day?' It is because they are only doing external Qigong, and are failing to practise the philosophy of Qigong.

Although their movements may be very beautiful and they may be able to sit or stand in meditation for over two hours, these people have not understood the philosophy of Qigong. It means their heart does not relate to their Qigong, so they cannot attain a very high level. It is a bit like some of the supermodels we see in fashion shows. Most people think they are very beautiful, but I can see that they are not so healthy. So even though someone may practise Qigong and their form looks good, if they do not practise with the right understanding and the right mental attitude (that is, the right heart), their skill will be limited.

To understand the philosophy behind Qigong, we must first understand that life is up and down. No experience is 100 per cent good or

100 per cent bad. Most of us can handle the good times even without Qigong practise, but it is the bad times that present the challenge. During times of emotional stress and physical problems, we definitely need proper Qigong practise to help us cope.

The first principle of practising Qigong is to be calm and relaxed. Most people find this very hard because it means changing how you think about things. Western society teaches us that when something happens to us, we should respond or act. Actually, this is not always necessary and can even cause more problems. Instead, we should first relax and calm ourselves. Then we should look at the situation clearly. Only when we are calm and our mind is clear should we think about the next step.

I know many people will disagree with me and think that taking no action is wrong. But Daoism says, 'Use stillness to deal with all things changing.' No response is actually a type of response in itself. Sometimes reacting will cause more conflict. If we are upset and then take it out on someone else, that person will also react. Their response will likely make us even more upset, because we have dealt with the problem emotionally rather than thinking about the end result. Therefore we should always keep ourselves calm and relaxed. That is the philosophy of Qigong.

Letting it all go

Recently I saw a documentary about a man in Singapore. He had his own business where he worked very hard. One day he found out that he had cancer, and the doctor told him he only had six months to live. He had always studied Buddhism, but not all that seriously. Now that he had only six months to live, he decided to give up his business and devote himself only to studying Buddhism.

In Buddhist education, he learned these principles: 'No wanting, no stubbornness, no classification' (that is, no thinking that one person or thing is better than another). Trying to follow these principles, he became more relaxed and let go a lot. His mind became calm and he did not worry about things. He even decided to stop taking his medical treatment, both Western and Chinese, and just follow nature and study more Buddhism. After six months he went back to see his doctor. The doctor was very surprised: the cancer cells had been greatly reduced. After one year, all the cancer cells had completely disappeared.

This is not a miracle. This makes perfect sense once you know how illness comes about. When people have cancer, it is because something in the body changes, becoming abnormal. If you want to go back to normal, then we must look at those things we are doing or thinking, or those things in our environment which have affected us.

The gentleman in Singapore completely let go of all his stress and worry. He began to eat more healthily and follow the Buddhist education, which advocates letting go instead of trying to hold on. The more we hold on to things like jealousy, worry, anger, greed or yearning, the more stress we make for ourselves. If it continues, this stress will cause the normal functioning of the body to change. The internal organs may not have enough Qi to cope and so things will start to break down. Eventually, illness will set in.

One of the other things this man learned in his studies was to help more people. In this way he forgot his own worries, which freed his mind. He did a lot of good things which meant that, eventually, more people helped him. This is cause and effect; when you can help others, you also feel good. When we feel good, then the body will respond accordingly. Without him even realising it, his body started to change to get better. When you see him now, you would never believe that he has had cancer. His face is very shiny and he is very happy and settled.

Cancer today is becoming more and more common. There is so much radiation in the environment, from satellites, mobile phones and computers. Our food is no longer natural, with so much of it genetically modified or with the nutritional value reduced through intensive farming. We are exposed to pollution every day. Even the chemicals from our household cleaning agents threaten our health if we do not do something to get rid of the toxins. Fasting and detoxifying can help, but they do not make your Qi stronger, and this is most important. When our Qi is strong, we can fight illness better. Qigong helps to make the immune system stronger.

Human technology is like a cancer in nature. If we put a halt to all these unnatural things, air quality would improve, the soil would recover and the water would become pure. All the trees, animals and human beings would become healthier. Ancient people often lived to be 100 years old. This was because they followed nature, living simple lives. They ate according to their climate and the season. They went to bed when it was dark and rose when it was light. They did not try to live outside of nature. They practised calmness, and did not easily become upset over small things.

When you practise Qigong, the best way to do it is to let go without trying to get a result. The less you want, the more you will get. If you can apply this philosophy, it can help you to become a better person. The more Qigong you practise, and the more you let go, then the more you will be able to achieve a high level of skill, and not only help yourself but help others. With this approach you will become calmer, more accepting, and you'll find that you are working on your heart, or attitude, as well as your body when you practise Qigong.

I would like to share one of my favourite Chinese stories with you. It was written a long time ago and is a true story about two scholars on their way to take the Imperial exams. The following story tells us how our actions create a certain result, for good or bad. It is all up to us.

TWO SCHOLARS

Once upon a time in Xinye County, Hunan Province, China, there was a temple known as the Jade Emperor Temple. It was quite far away from town, but many people still liked to visit it. The temple was very popular as it made a lot of people's wishes come true.

One day, two young scholars, Zhang and Li, were on their way to the capital to take the Imperial Examination and they decided to visit Jade Emperor Temple before they went on to the capital. At that time, the Chinese government held this special examination every four years in order to find the most talented people to help them run the country. If they passed with high marks, then they would be very famous in the whole country and earn a lot of respect from other people and be able to get a good position.

Zhang and Li came to the temple. Inside was a table behind which stood a Daoist named Ci Hui. On the table he had a sign which read,

'Your date tells your life and death. My prediction tells your good and bad. I can save you, if you believe me.'

The two young men looked at the sign and then looked at the Daoist and then said to each other, 'He does not look like an ordinary man. He looks like an Immortal! Maybe he can tell us our future as we are going for the Imperial Examinations.'

Although they were strangers, the two young gentlemen sat down at the Daoist's table together and asked Ci Hui if he could tell their fortunes. First, he asked for Zhang's date of birth and looked at his face. Then he started to do some calculations on his fingers and murmuring certain words as he touched the pad of each finger with his thumb. This is actually a traditional way to find out the Five Elements for the hour, day, month and year of birth of a person's horoscope.

He then looked at Zhang and said, 'Congratulations! You will pass tomorrow's Imperial Examination with high marks. You are in luck. This is because in your last life, you did a lot of good things and you are going to be rewarded in this life.' Of course, Zhang was very happy to hear this. He bowed to the old man and paid him and then left to go back to the place where he was staying.

Next the old Daoist looked at Li and did the same calculations and looked at his face. After a few moments, he said to Li, 'I am sorry, but your fortune is not good. In fact, it is very bad. Forget taking the Imperial Examination because today you are going to die. You have this ill fate because in your last life you did a lot of bad things and so now must pay back.'

Li was shocked. He felt all his Qi leave his body and his face become pale. He paid Ci Hui and stumbled from the temple in a daze, feeling his whole life turn upside down.

Zhang, on the other hand, was so full of happy spirits that he was like one in a good dream. He wandered here and there enjoying the scenery around him. He suddenly arrived at a rope bridge that crossed a powerful river. The bridge was not that stable and only had loose wooden planks as a walkway. As Zhang was crossing over, he accidentally kicked some of the planks and they dropped into the river, leaving a big gap. He guiltily looked around to see if anyone had seen what he did. When he saw that no one had, he turned quickly to run away. However, as he

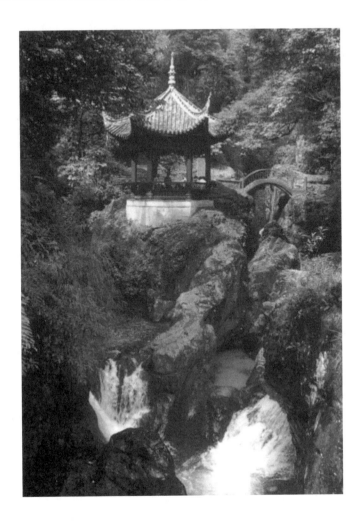

ran back up the pathway, in his hurry he knocked over an old man who was coming around the bend in the path. He did not think about helping the old man up, but continued to run.

Li had been also walking and he came to the bridge from the opposite side. He was very depressed. As he walked across the bridge, he was so lost in his thoughts that he almost fell into the gap left by the missing planks. The gap was big enough that he could easily have fallen through if he had not caught himself in time. He stood gasping on the bridge with his heart beating fast.

Just then, he looked up to see an old man coming towards him on the other side of the gap. Li thought about what Ci Hui had told him. If he was going to die today, he thought he would try and do something good and maybe atone for some of the bad things he had done in his previous lifetimes. So he called out to help the old man.

He shouted, 'Sir, be careful, there is a gap here. You should turn and go back! Don't come this way!'

The old man replied, 'But I must go across here as I have to go to my home. My old wife is waiting for me. There is no other way. I am sure that I will be able to find some way to cross.'

Li thought for a moment and then said, 'OK, how about this. I will lie down and cover the gap and then you can walk over me.'

The old man was very impressed by this and he was able to cross over the gap. He started praising Li for his goodness when suddenly it started to pour down with rain. Li took off his coat and covered the old man and helped him the rest of the way to his home. The old man said to Li, 'You are a good-hearted person. You must have a good future ahead of you. Live long and take care.'

Li decided to find a hotel to hide himself in, hoping to avoid any bad fortune that might be the cause of his death. After the dinner, Li went to bed and covered himself with the blanket, waiting to see if he would be able to pass the night alive. Eventually, after much worrying, he fell asleep without even realising it. The next day, he was so surprised when he woke to find the sun shining in his face. He was not dead! He was so excited that he hurried to pay his bill and go back to the Jade Temple to see Ci Hui.

He walked into the temple and saw the old Daoist, the same as yesterday. He was sitting very straight in his chair, his hands folded as if he was waiting for him. Ci Hui said to Li, 'Good morning, Mr Li. It is good to see you again. Today, your face is in luck.'

Li said, 'Sifu, I don't understand. Yesterday you said I was going to die and yet today you say I am lucky. How can this be?'

Ci Hui laughed loudly. He said, 'You must have done some good things yesterday. Maybe you did something to help someone else, thinking about more about their well-being than your own. These good deeds changed your fate.'

The Old Daoist then leaned over the table and clapped his hand on Li's shoulder and said with a great smile, 'Hurry up and go to the capital to take the Imperial Examination! You will place number one!' So Li hurried off to do as he was bid.

After some weeks, the results of the examination were announced, and it came about that Li had, indeed, won first place. He received much attention and praise and became very famous throughout the country. However, Zhang did not place at all and did not get any title. Upset, Zhang went back to the Jade Emperor Temple to talk to the old Daoist.

He saw Ci Hui sitting in his usual place and he knelt before him and asked, 'Sifu, when I came to visit you before, you said I was very lucky and that I would come first in the examinations. However, I did not place at all. Why is this?'

Ci Hui said to Zhang, 'Ask yourself, what did you do in the time before the examination to change your fate?' He then told Zhang to look at the statue of the Jade Emperor behind him. When Zhang did this, his face went pale. The face of the statue was the exact image of the old man whom he had knocked down that day by the bridge.

Watching Zhang, Ci Hui said, 'Sometimes we think no one sees our actions. However, all our actions will eventually have their result.'

This is a very good story. There is no person who is perfectly good and there is no person who is perfectly bad. The more good deeds you do, the more good results you get. The more bad deeds you do, the more bad results you get. When we practise Qigong, it is the same. If we practise with the right heart and also do more good things in our life, then we can reach a high level of expertise in Qigong.

Yin and Yang

CHINESE PHILOSOPHY is based upon balance. We believe that in any situation, under any circumstance or with any new development, that balance is the most important thing. When things are balanced, they will bring good results that will last until something happens to change things. So the longer you can keep things balanced, the better results you will get and the longer things will last. For example, from time to time, you need to balance the wheels of your car, as otherwise your tyres will get damaged. The same is true with walking. You have to keep your weight and your movements balanced, as this will make the hip joints more flexible and take away any stress from the spine. If you are too tense or your posture is incorrect, you will end up hurting your back.

In Chinese philosophy, balance can help things to grow. But to have balance, we have to have two equal sides. One side we call Yin and the other side is Yang. As we saw in Chapter 1, Yin encompasses passive qualities – dark, soft, feminine, slow, or the night, the moon, etc. Yang encompasses active qualities – bright, hard, masculine, fast, or the day, the sun, etc.

We often see Yin and Yang portrayed as in the Taiji symbol (see page 26). *Tai* means big and *Ji* means limited. The dark part represents Yin and the light part represents Yang. However, one thing you should not forget is that Yin and Yang need a middle line to balance them. You could say this line separates Yin and Yang, but it is just as correct to say that it is also the connection between them. This particular symbol shows us that within everything Yin, there is some Yang and within everything Yang, there is some Yin. It also shows us that when something comes to its fullest point, it will change into its opposite. We can see this with the decline of Yin merging with the fullest part of Yang and vice versa.

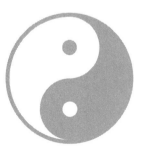

Once a student asked me, 'Why do we always see the Yin and Yang symbol like this? Can we draw different symbols?' The answer is yes, you can draw the symbol in many different ways (see below).

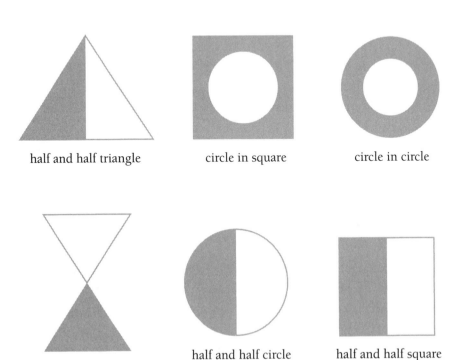

half and half triangle

circle in square

circle in circle

two triangles

half and half circle

half and half square

In Chinese philosophy, we believe that to go too far forward is not good and also to go too far backward is not good. In the past, people in China were not educated to be the best or number one. Instead, they were taught that being the second, third or even fourth or fifth best was preferable. The reason behind this is that taking anything to its extreme will inevitably mean it will bounce back, sooner rather than later.

Let me give you an example. During the Qing Dynasty (1644–1912 AD), there was a man named Zeng Guo Fan. He did a lot for the Qing government and was promoted to a very high position within it. At this time, even though they were a minority, the Manchurians ruled the whole of China. It has to be remembered that in China then, as today, there were many different ethnic groups. The major groups are the Manchurians, Mongolians, Wui, Han and Tibetans, but there are also many other smaller ethnic groups.

The Han people were the largest group, but during the Qing Dynasty, they were treated like second or third-class citizens by the Manchurians. However, Zeng Guo Fan was something of an exception. A Han, he was promoted to the highest position a Han person could hold. He was also insightful and could see that things were going to the extreme, so he decided to let go of a lot of his money and his position. He even gave his library the name 'Wish to be Broken'. He did all this because he knew that it was not good to go too far. He also knew that after things are good, the bad times will come. Of course, after the bad times, then good will come again. This is natural and balanced. This is Yin and Yang.

Today, I find that science misses this balance and might be going too far. We like to think we know so much more, but for me, today's scientific ideas for healing have not even reached the level of what already existed thousands of years ago in China. Chinese people already knew how to perform surgery, using only acupuncture as an anaesthestic. However, they found that it was a crude way to try and fix the problem. Instead, they began to develop how to diagnose, heal and balance the body without having to resort to this kind of radical invasion. They instead used herbs, acupuncture, massage, exercise and diet therapy to restore harmony to the body.

From my own experience, I have seen many people who have had surgery for a knee or shoulder problem. However, instead of getting better, more stiffness is created because all the channels, which are pathways for Qi, have been damaged. Until the body can create a new pathway for the Qi to go through, then the injury will not heal.

A question of balance

In Traditional Chinese Medicine, a doctor will try to find out what has caused the blockage in the joints, creating stiffness or pain. Joint pain is related to circulation and the correct function of the liver. In Chinese medicine, it is believed that every illness can be treated and that there is no incurable disease. It is the same for Qigong. If both Yin and Yang are balanced in the body, then we will have harmony and health.

By contrast, the Western concept of medicine is concerned only with how to cure an illness or treat the symptoms of pain. However, in so many cases, it is the medicine or the treatment that will kill the patient, not the disease. My own father was given so many different kinds of medication and treatments for his heart problem that, in the end, they made his condition worse and caused his kidneys to fail. Chinese medicine knows that for the heart to be healthy, then the kidneys need to be healthy and so they will try to make the kidneys stronger to help the other problems.

Using the Yin/Yang theory, we know that when the body has too much heat, we need to cool it down. When the body has too much heat, it can mean the kidneys are weak and not producing enough water, allowing too much fire to get too strong and so affect the heart. To restore balance, the heat needs to be released or cooled down. Chinese people will use movement, food or herbs to cool it down and will try to bring up the strength of the weaker, internal organs.

Meanwhile, Western medicine keeps doing more research to look for cures for disease and drugs and vaccines to kill or protect against new illnesses. From this you can tell it is a never-ending cycle that will not have a clear solution. It is like someone who does not have a job, yet keeps borrowing money from the bank to pay his bills.

Chinese medicine does not think solely about attacking, isolating and finding the cure for one disease. It looks instead at the individual and the whole body. This is why, traditionally, a medicine is made up to suit the individual and their body type and condition. There can be many factors that cause the same disease, not just one. Additionally, some people may have a weak spleen and so cannot take certain herbs that another person can take to heal the same problem. A good Chinese doctor will adjust the prescription to match the person and try to restore the balance of Yin and Yang in the body.

In addition to restoring balance to the body, Chinese medicine also considers how to make the body stronger so that it can adapt to all kinds of situations. If someone becomes ill, the way to heal the illness is to strengthen the internal organs by making the Qi in the body stronger.

If you develop a disease, this means that there is a weakness somewhere in the body that has laid it open to attack. The way to fight the problem is to strengthen the affected part, instead of trying to kill the virus or create a vaccine against the germ. It is not so much the virus that causes the problem as finding any weakness in yourself and whether your Qi is strong enough to overcome the problem. In Qigong, we do movement to help open the channels so that Qi can flow. If Qi cannot flow, the body cannot get stronger. This is using positive Yang to overcome negative Yin.

So in the case of someone needing money, the best thing for them to do is to find a job and work for it rather than borrow it. In other words, when a person is ill, they need to strengthen the body so it can handle the job of healing by itself, rather than always need to borrow the means for healing from another source. Borrowing 'money' still does not get rid of the problem and can even create more of a problem.

I often think of medicine as a big tree. If the leaves have a problem, Western physicians will try to treat each leaf. A practitioner of TCM will try to treat the roots of the tree instead.

The 2003 SARS epidemic in Asia is a good example of this. Why did some people survive and others did not? For me, it is because some people's Qi was strong enough to fight the illness while that of others was not. The government found some animals that had the SARS virus, but their bodies also had an antibody to balance it and so they could still survive even though they had the virus. Actually, this is the way Qigong and Chinese medicine works. It makes the Qi strong, so that even though a person may have cancer, it cannot go too far to attack the body.

Essentially, the more drugs we take, the less we rely on nature and ourselves to heal the body. The body should be able to balance itself and create its own defences to fight any problems. The more we rely on outside things, the weaker our immune system will get. For myself, I always say that Qigong is my medicine.

In many ways, people living in the last century were healthier physically, because they were far more active. People did not live as long, but they were able to do most things. Today, some people live a long time, but in old age cannot take care of themselves and have to have help even for dressing and eating. If we keep trying to produce all these artificial ways to prolong life and keep going against the balance of nature, eventually we will not be able to go on. It would be good if science and technology slowed down so that we can live on this planet a bit longer and in a fit state to enjoy it.

Playing the fool to regain harmony

There is a Chinese saying, 'Being a fool is not bad.' And sometimes this is true. For instance, if you act like a fool, your enemies will not pay too much attention to you, and so you are safer. Science today is very clever, being able to dissect even the smallest cells and change DNA, however, the end result might not be so good. Just because we *can* do something, does not mean that we *should* do it.

There is a story about a very smart man who lived during the Spring and Autumn Period (8th–5th century BC) who actually pretended to be crazy so that he could escape from being held hostage. His name was Sun Bin. He had a friend named Peng Juan. There were both very good at strategy. Although Peng Juan was good, his classmate, Sun Bin, was even better. They both studied under the same teacher, Gui Guizi, who was also very famous and knew a great deal about all sorts of things. When Sun Bin and Peng Juan finished their studies with their teacher, they both went back to their own countries, China not being unified at this time.

Peng Juan had a very good position in the government of Wei. He invited his classmate, Sun Bin, to come to visit him and maybe help him in the government. Sun Bin was good in politics, strategy, prediction, using the *Yijing* and understanding about people. The King of Wei liked Sun Bin very much, so much that eventually Peng Juan got jealous. So Peng Juan had him arrested and then crippled him, branded his face and kept him in a house with spies to watch over him because he did not want Sun Bin to take away his place with the King.

However, Sun Bin pretended that he had gone mad and acted crazy. He laughed when he should have cried and cried when he should have laughed, and talked nothing but nonsense. He wanted Peng Juan to believe he had gone crazy so he would relax his guard and think him harmless. His plan worked, and it gave Sun Bin the chance to escape back to his own country, Qi, where he was highly respected by the ruling king there. In the end, the King of Qi knew Sun Bin was very accomplished and asked him to help rule his country.

So sometimes it is good to act a little dumb or foolish if it means you can keep balance in your life.

Qigong practise also needs balance. I have come across many people who do a lot of movement but no meditation. They end up sustaining injuries, particularly in their joints. Some people, on the other hand, do a lot of meditation and no movement, but this makes their bodies weak and they do not have enough strength to get through the day easily. For our health to stay balanced, we need both the movement and meditation. This covers both Yin and Yang and will make us healthy.

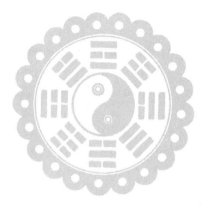

CHAPTER

5 Five Elements

Cʜɪɴᴇꜱᴇ ᴄᴏɴꜱɪᴅᴇʀ that everything in the universe has a special kind of energy. In the last chapter we talked about Yin and Yang, which is the energy of opposites. There is also a special kind of universal energy which can be classified into five different types of energies called 'elements'. These Five Elements are water, fire, wood, earth and metal. In fact, along with the Yin/Yang theory, the theory of the Five Elements is the basis of all Chinese culture, including Feng Shui, astrology, traditional medicine, Qigong and even diet.

Development of the Five Elements

The idea of the Five Elements is founded upon many thousands of years of observation of both earth and heaven. In ancient China, the society was an agricultural one as far back as 7,000 years. The people were very primitive then. Their lives were completely dependent upon the changing of the seasons and good weather for planting, growing and harvesting their food. Many times they did not have enough food because there was famine or flooding. Over time, they tried to find some way in which they could predict whether a year would be good or bad. They would heat certain animal bones until they cracked and then a special person would read the cracks and lines made by the heat to find out whether there would be good or bad luck.

Later, during the Xia Dynasty (21 BC), the method of prediction was improved. It included knowledge of the stars in the sky, observations of the sun and moon and further development of the Chinese calendar. This calendar divided the year into five seasons, including spring, summer, late summer, autumn and winter. From these five seasons, many observations were made about the development of the Five Elements of wood, water, fire, earth and metal.

These ancient people also saw that many other things around them were related and could be classified according to the Five Elements. Each element had a flavour, a grain and a sound to which it related. They found that people had five emotions, five internal organs and five sense organs. These all connected with the five seasons and the energies that they brought as the cycles of the earth and heaven changed.

For instance, spring was a time of growing and renewal. It was when the sun warmed the soil so that plants could begin to grow, so they called this a 'wood' season. Summer was hot in middle China and so it became associated with heat and fire. Late summer is a special season and was a filling-in time which bridged between summer and autumn. It could be both hot and cool and was the centre of the seasons. Therefore, this was associated with earth, a time when the fullness of summer was beginning to change.

Autumn was a time of harvesting and of sunset. At this time, metal containers for cooking and storage had already been created. This metal was the harvest of the earth. Therefore earth became associated with the element metal. Winter was a time of cold and snow, both of which were forms of water. Therefore winter was related to the water element.

These five seasons also related to the directions of the compass. However, China draws the directions of the compass opposite to the West. East will be on the left, representing the rising sun. As the sun rises, it becomes very hot, so instead of south being at the bottom, we put south at the top of the compass because heat rises. West is on the right side, showing the setting of the sun. Water will seek the lowest point and so runs downwards. That is why north is at the bottom. We know that the Five Elements relate to five directions, not just four, so the last direction is the centre and relates to earth. It was from this stable point that all these observations could be made. Without a base or a centre,

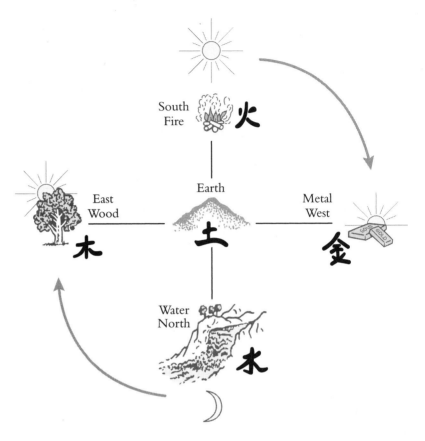

you would not be able to find your direction. This centre is like the Dantian in our body, where all things develop.

This Five Element theory, combined with understanding of Yin and Yang, is the foundation of all things in Chinese culture. This simplicity and unified thinking is why Chinese culture has lasted so many thousands of years. Chinese knowledge follows the same principle no matter whether you are a musician, scholar, emperor or ordinary person.

By contrast, knowledge in the West is based upon so many different theories. If you are a musician, you probably know very little about science. Scientists do not know anything about medicine unless they particularly study it. In the West, any subject must be studied individually. But in China, once you understand the underlying principle of one thing, it applies to all kinds of skills. At the highest level, all skill is the same.

For example, a farmer may not know how to do Chinese calligraphy, but they will be able to tell if the calligraphy is good or not. This is because they are able to see the energy and flow of the writing. A farmer lives closely with the seasons and nature. In the past, they could look at the sky and know the weather and could look at the soil and tell if it was ready to plant. They could predict the outcome for so many things just by observing certain things around them.

By observing animals and the people around them, they could see human nature very clearly. So although they might not know how to write or even read calligraphy, they still could see the character of a person's writing. They could see whether or not the person was calm or passionate or whether they were powerful, like a general. If the calligraphy was fine and organised, they knew that the writer was a gentleman, like a scholar. All these personalities were like the five emotions, five seasons and five tastes which were part of their daily life.

SUPPORT AND CONTROL

There is a special relationship between all of the Five Elements. Each element has another element that gives it support and nourishment. In the supporting cycle, wood nourishes fire; fire makes earth; earth creates metal; metal attracts water; water nourishes wood. This is also called the Five Element creation or helping cycle (see below).

Five Elements: Creating Cycle

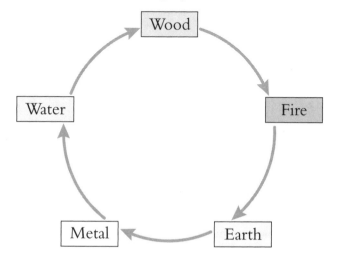

If we know Yin and Yang theory, then we know that if there is a supporting element, then there must also be an element that controls and takes energy away. In the controlling cycle, metal cuts wood; wood takes the nutrients from earth; earth stops water; water extinguishes fire and fire melts metal (see below). Understanding the relationship of the elements in both the supporting and controlling cycle will help you to understand all aspects of Chinese culture and also help you to balance your life and health.

Five Elements: Controlling Cycle

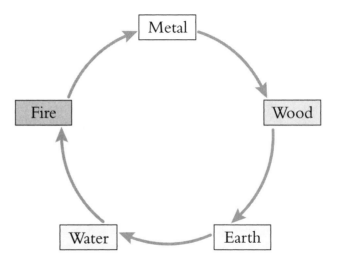

FENG SHUI

For Feng Shui, the Five Elements show us how to balance the different energies of the universe so we can make our home harmonious or office prosperous. Each year the directions from which the energy for good luck, money, ceremony, sickness and bad luck come change.

Once we know the directions from which these energies come, we can use the inter-relationship of the Five Elements to bring up the positive energy and release or control the negative energy.

HOROSCOPES AND PERSONALITY

For horoscopes, this same principle is used. Because the Five Elements also relate to certain times of the hour, day, month and year, we can find out to which element our personality relates. We do this by looking at the day element. There is a special Chinese almanac that is used to calculate this. Once we know our day element, we can know more about our personality traits and our talents.

For instance, if you are wood element, then it means you will like nature, even gardening. You will like to be outdoors a lot, are artistic and like to create things. A fire person is active, charming and will like to talk a lot. They will stand out in a group as they have a lot of Yang energy. On the other hand, an earth person likes studying and reading and will be very patient for things. A water person is easy-going and very sociable with lots of friends. A metal person is organised and is good for planning things. They are very loyal and can sometimes be really stubborn.

Some people may find that they have the characteristics of more than one element, but usually there will be one dominant element. Knowing our element means we can learn how to balance ourselves with others. For instance, we can see from the above charts that metal attracts water. If you are a metal person, then you will find that you will feel comfortable with and attract water element people.

Sometimes, though, you may find that you meet someone who always tries to control you or who makes you feel uncomfortable. This means your elements are not in harmony. Maybe you are wood and the other person is metal. We know in the Five Element theory that metal cuts wood. This means metal controls wood but this does not mean that we should avoid that person. Instead we can use the Five Element theory to balance the situation. Although the wood element does not like to face the metal element, even a sharp knife has a dull side. So you can try to avoid the sharp side of that person's personality. It is better to make a friend than an enemy. If we want to set a good example for living peacefully, then this is the wise choice.

Chinese say, 'A broken mouth does not like to see a broken bowl.' It is true that no one likes to be reminded of their own shortcomings or weaknesses. However, when we feel uncomfortable with someone, we should try to learn from the situation and then we can also understand ourselves and others better.

FIVE ELEMENTS AND PERSONALITY

Together, these cycles create complete balance and harmony. We can use the Five Elements to tell a lot of things, even about someone's personality and their health. For instance, if we say someone is a 'wood person', this means that they might like gardening or being outdoors in nature a lot, like the colour green and is artistic.

A fire person is active, talkative, very charming. They will stand out in a group, as they are full of energy. An earth person likes studying and reading. They are quite patient and are quieter. A metal person likes everything in order, so they will be good for filing and organising things. A water person is easy-going, has a good heart, likes to help out with things and is sociable.

We can see that we may have more than one Five Element characteristic, but usually there will be one that is the main one and which we belong to more than the others. Using the Five Element charts above, then you can see what kind of person you will attract and be attracted to by looking at which element supports or nourishes your element.

FIVE ELEMENTS AND INTERNAL ORGANS

The Five Elements relate to more than personality, however. They also correspond to our health and the internal organs. Wood relates to the liver and gall bladder. Fire relates to the heart and small intestine. Earth relates to the spleen and stomach. Metal relates to the lungs and large intestine. Water relates to the kidneys and bladder. These organs have special functions in the body and also have corresponding emotions which relate to them.

In TCM theory, the liver is seen as creating and governing the blood, so if someone has poor circulation, this means their liver is weak. In Five Element theory, the liver is related to wood and in the creation cycle we know that water nourishes wood. We also know that water relates to the kidneys, so if we make the kidneys stronger, we can support the liver.

In Healthy Living Gong, we can also use the Five Element theory to help us choose the right exercise to work on a specific problem. So to make the liver stronger, we can do *Collecting Qi to the Dantian*. If you want to make your kidneys stronger, then you can do *Old Tree with Winding Roots* and *Looking for Treasure at the Bottom of the Chest*.

Another example is if you have a stomach problem. The stomach and spleen relate to the earth element. In most cases, stomach problems are from too much stomach acid. This means we need to release, instead of support, the earth element. So the element which helps to release some of the earth energy is metal. This is because earth creates metal and is like a mother pregnant with her child. The child will take the mother's energy and she will find her body weaker.

The Five Element theory is actually very simple, but in the beginning it is difficult for many people as they do not understand the relationships of the elements. When you understand this theory well, you will understand everything in life. You will understand Chinese medicine, and you will understand why people act the way they do. Even each hour, day, month and year has its own element so you can understand why some days go smoothly (based on your element and the element of the day) and some go not so smoothly. When we understand this, then we can let go and accept this is nature and not be upset by so many small things.

Qigong

The Five Elements of our bodies are left, right, front and back and centre. The centre is our Dantian. *Dan* means crystal and *Tian* means field. We can see from the special name that it is a very important part of our body, this is where our Qi is stored. If we do not store the Qi that we gather from our Qigong practise, then we will not build up a reserve supply to have when we get ill. Our extra Qi is like having savings in the bank in case of an emergency.

When we have enough Qi, then our bodies feel good and even if we become ill, we have enough Qi to help us fight the illness so that we can recover. The more we practise Qigong, then the more Qi we can store. However, if we do not have enough Qi stored in the Dantian, then it is much harder to recover from illness. When we are ill, we use Qigong to make our Qi stronger.

In Qigong, we can also use our knowledge of the Five Elements to help strengthen particular internal organs. If we practise facing the south, this relates to the heart and will bring up the fire energy. If we practise facing the north, this relates to kidneys. East is for liver, west is for the lungs and centre is for the spleen.

If we understand more about the Five Elements, which one is supporting and which one is controlling, then we know how to balance our health, our diet and our actions.

The principle of the Five Elements is to help you balance yourself in any situation. I have talked more about the health side of the Five Elements in Chapter 8, 'How Palms and Face Relate to Health'.

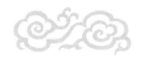

When and How to Practise Qigong

6

I AM OFTEN ASKED when is the best time to practise Qigong. Usually I say twice a day: practise in the morning and in the evening. People seem to accept this answer, but surprisingly they do not ask me why.

As a teacher, I think a lot about the best way to help my students. I think most teachers, if they have been teaching long enough, will usually have a method for making things very simple for beginners who do not know much about the subject. We will give them a very simple answer. When they have been studying for longer and have a certain level of knowledge, then you will teach them differently, and you may even contradict some things you taught or said to them earlier.

Do you know why this happens? It's to prevent confusion in the beginner. We want them to be able to build up a good foundation and understanding of the principles. If we explain too much in the beginning, they will become very confused and think that the subject is very difficult. This might cause them to give up or lose interest.

This is how children were taught in old times in China. Old times refer to the time from the Han Dynasty in 206 BC to the Qing Dynasty, which ended in AD 1911 and refers to a way of teaching that was used for over a thousand years. Primary schools usually had only 10 to 15 children aged from seven to 12 years old. During this period, they would study Confucianism (Ru Jia), the philosophy of the 6th-century thinker Confucius. (His real name was Kong Fu Zi. Confucius is an accepted

Westernisation of his name.) This is because it taught people how to be respectable and good. So the first thing children learned was how to be a good person, so when they grew up they would be useful in society.

Children of this age were still too young to understand all the meanings of the things they were studying. They read all the Confucian books and learned them off by heart so they could recite them with their teacher. However, nothing was explained. When the teacher read a sentence, they would repeat it and also learn how to write it. When they reached the age of 12, they would be able to recite all the Confucian books by heart without referring back to the original text. They would then go to *Tai Sher*, the equivalent of university. In old China, there were no secondary or high schools. However, the teacher would take the students to different places, almost like a holiday. The teacher would then explain all the meanings of what they had studied by relating the ideas to nature, people and even the government of the day, and then he would ask them questions about what they had learned.

Today, education is very different. We concentrate on technology, mathematics, science, history and grammar. There is nothing taught on how to be a good person in the society. People today think that when you talk about how to behave, you are talking about religion. However, in China, this teaching about good behaviour was a way of making society balanced so that it would last longer. If everyone in society only thought about themselves and not about how to help each other, many people would have died. Families depended on each other and children took care of their parents in old age in the same way the parents cared for the children when they were babies.

Personally, I think this method is a very good one. So when teaching beginners, I use the method they used in ancient China and give them very simple answers, and help them understand the basics of Qigong.

When I recommend practising Qigong twice a day, this is general advice for the beginner. Daytime is Yang, because when the sun comes up the energy is active. In the evening, when the sun goes down, the energy is calmer and Yin. If we can balance both of nature's energies, active and calm, Yin and Yang, then we can become part of nature. So nature will help us to balance ourselves, give us good Qi and release negative Qi. Later, when you understand more about Qi, you will find that all times are good for practising Qigong, from midnight to the next midnight, and that there are even special times which stimulate a particular organ or channel in the body.

A different clock

In the past, the Chinese did not keep time by following a 24-hour clock. Instead, they had twelve hours often referred to as the Chinese Animal Hours (see below). Traditionally every two hours on the Western clock counts as one Chinese hour. In China, these 'hours' have special names and so if, say, you were born during the Zi hour, then people would know that you were born during the time of 11pm–1am. It might also be referred to as the hour of the rat, because each of these hours also corresponds to the twelve Chinese animal signs that are used in horoscopes.

ANIMALS AND THE HOURS

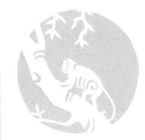

Hours	Animals	Channels
11pm–1am	Rat	Gall Bladder
1–3am	Ox	Liver
3–5am	Tiger	Lung
5–7am	Rabbit	Large Intestine
7–9am	Dragon	Stomach
9–11am	Snake	Spleen
11am–1pm	Horse	Heart
1–3pm	Sheep	Small Intestine
3–5pm	Monkey	Urinary Bladder
5–7pm	Rooster	Kidney
7–9pm	Dog	Pericardium
9–11pm	Pig	Sanjiao

In addition, you can see from the above chart that each hour also helps different channels in the body. They also relate to many more things as well, like months and different directions. However, we are most interested in how these hours can help us in our Qigong practise.

When we practise Qigong at a certain time, this means that there is a certain energy that is present in nature that will benefit a particular internal organ. So when you wake up in the morning and start to practise your Qigong, your stomach will benefit. After you have finished work, go home and have your dinner and start to practise at 7pm, then your heart will benefit, as the pericardium relates to the heart. By practising at these times, you will benefit both your stomach and your heart. If you have two healthy internal organs, then other organs will benefit and become healthy as well, so you do not need to think that you have to practise all of the twelve hours of each day.

Most people will practise in the morning and evening. However, when you have more time, you might want to practise three times a day. So you can choose a third time, such as 10am, as then your small intestine and digestive system will also benefit. If you are really short on time, though, and can only practise once a day after work, you will still benefit.

It is very simple. The more you practise, the more you will benefit. It is a very simple formula, like one plus one equals two. Some people will try to practise maybe two or even three hours and afterwards they will feel more tired than when they started. This is not right.

You should feel good and have more energy after your practise. If you feel tired, it is because you are *using* energy rather than gathering energy in your practise. Let me explain. If you have been ill or have never done any Qigong practise, then maybe even 10 or 15 minutes is a long time for you. So try to practise morning and evening for that amount of time. Then if you want to do longer, you can build up gradually. Usually people will use a lot of energy in their work and so even if they have practised in the morning, they will have used the Qi that they gathered and stored. That is why I suggest another session before going to bed. This will help bring the body back to normal.

However, the most important thing is yourself. It is best to find a time when you can practise consistently. That way you will get into the habit and it will become your routine. Today, people are so busy and try so many things but they never carry on long enough to develop their skills. There's a Chinese saying, '*Geen yat bo, han yat bo*', which means 'Look one step, walk one step.' If you just let your Qi develop naturally without wanting too much, you will find you can carry on longer. I do not mean longer as in practising two hours instead of one. What I mean is, practising for a lifetime rather than one month or one year.

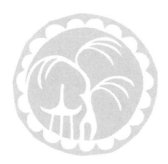

7 Breathing

BREATHING IS VERY important in Qigong, so how do we breathe when we do Qigong?

I have met people who have asked me whether they should breathe in through the nose and out through the mouth or should they breathe from the abdomen. Some ask whether or not we should take as deep a breath as possible when we breathe. Others want to know if we should think about Qi (energy).

These are all different types of breathing, but which one is best? My suggestion is that you try all three of the breathing methods below. You can try at home, but you should try each method for at least between five and 15 minutes, because if the time is any shorter, you will not be able to see any difference. See how you feel and see how you should breathe, either through the nose or mouth or both.

1. Breathe in through the nose and out through the nose.

2. Breathe in through the nose and out through the mouth.

3. Breathe in through the mouth and out through the mouth.

After you have tried this small experiment, I think that you will find that breathing in and out through the nose is easier and you stay more relaxed. When you breathe either in or out through your mouth, you will find that you can become tired and some people might feel dizzy.

You will see that it will feel uncomfortable and not natural to breathe like this for more than five or 10 minutes. You will also find you cannot breathe with your mouth for more than five minutes. This is because the mouth is meant for eating and talking.

If the mouth were meant for breathing, it would have been designed quite differently. Instead of taste buds and saliva glands, which only work well when the mouth is closed, the mouth would have the kind of built-in filtering system that the nose does, the tiny hairs that catch dust and pollution trying to enter the body. So if you remember the story of the little old lady who swallowed a fly, you know the moral of the story is to keep the mouth closed and breathe through the nose. Then you will not swallow flies!

However, when you breathe through the nose, you use as little effort as possible to take each breath. You can still breathe through your nose while you are talking, eating, moving and sleeping (though some people find this hard). But if you breathe through your mouth, you cannot do any of these things, apart from sleeping.

Breathing and Qi

When you are healthy, you have no problem with breathing through your nose. The air you breathe in will go to your lungs and the lungs will transform this as pure Qi which will nourish the body. When we breathe through the nose, the body and internal organs will be more relaxed and the breath and also the Qi will sink naturally to the Dantian.

Qi is the essence of the air we breathe. When Qi sinks to the Dantian, it means we are breathing from the abdomen, because the Dantian is here. This might sound odd or difficult; but as long as you relax your upper body, breathe through your nose and keep your mouth closed, you will automatically breathe with the Dantian, and the Qi will store there. In this instance, we are referring to the Lower Dantian. We actually have three Dantians in the body: the Lower Dantian (located just below the navel), the Middle Dantian (located at the Middle Chest), and the Upper Dantian (located at the forehead). Each Dantian has a particular function, the Lower Dantian storing the Qi gathered from our Qigong practise.

So as you practise Qigong, relax your chest and upper body and breathe naturally. If the upper body is not relaxed, the shoulders will be tense and the Qi will not sink to the Dantian. When we are under stress, the shoulders will become tense and tight, you find it difficult to breathe through your nose and Qi will not sink to the Dantian. The Dantian is like a safe where you store all your valuables. The most valuable thing your body can have is plenty of good Qi. It is the battery that keeps you healthy and helps you to live longer.

If you want to store more treasure, you have to open the safe to allow the treasure to go in. To open the safe, you need to relax the upper body – the chest, neck and all your muscles. If there is any stiffness, then the safe will close and you will not be able to get enough Qi to your Dantian. With a healthy person, the upper body is relaxed and the lower body is strong. Your arms do not need to be too strong, they just need a certain level of strength and that is enough.

Some people might find it difficult to breathe through the nose all the time. Even children today find it hard to do, particularly when they are running or doing physical training. This is because their lungs are weak. Asthma and hay fever, in fact, are very much on the increase. However, training more and breathing through the nose can really help these problems, while using medicines or inhalers all the time will only make the lungs weaker and the problem worse.

When I used to travel down to London every week, I found that during the summer months I suffered terribly from hay fever. My eyes would water, my nose would run and I would sneeze a lot. Still, I just kept going and would force myself to breathe through the nose as much as possible. When I found it difficult, I would just do more meditation. Now, six years later, I do not have any problems with hay fever, even in other countries where pollen is very bad.

So even if you find it too difficult to breathe through the nose and are tempted to go back to breathing through the mouth, try not to get into this habit. Remember that breathing through the mouth will make you lose Qi and will make you tired and can even affect your emotions, making you depressed and anxious.

Of course, when you are very ill there is often no way you can breathe through your nose all the time. So you can use the second method instead, breathe in through your nose and out through your mouth. This way, you can still store some Qi in your Dantian, although it is not ideal. This is because you will not be releasing enough of the old, negative Qi from your body. If you are very, very weak, and you can hardly breathe through your nose, then you have no choice but to breathe through your mouth. But you should remember you will store even less Qi and release even less negative Qi from the body.

In emergencies, too, breathing through the mouth is often necessary. If someone is injured very seriously and they have to go into hospital where they have a breathing tube put down their throat, then they cannot breathe through their nose. All they can do is try and relax the body and let the Qi flow inside the body better. Then they might be able to take a certain amount of energy in through the skin, and this will help. The right kind of food can also help give energy. However, if a person is highly traumatised, they will not even have enough energy to eat.

If you have been through a serious illness or shock, another way to help the body recover is to do some simple exercises to recharge your Qi. Even if you just do some stretching and meditation initially, it will help to make you stronger.

Therefore, the proper way to breathe and gather more Qi is to breathe in and out of the nose as much as possible, whether you are still or moving. The second way is to breathe in through the nose and out through the mouth, but only because you are too weak to do otherwise. The last way is to breathe both in and out through the mouth. In this way you will actually lose energy from the body, so if at all possible, you should try to avoid this.

You might have heard mentioned that when keeping the mouth closed, the tip of the tongue should touch the upper palette at the back of the top teeth. Actually, when you close your mouth, your tongue will automatically be in this position as there is no other place it can go (unless you are very unusual).

Some people may talk about using visualisation to direct the breathing, such as imagining the Qi coming up the *Du Mai* (back channel) as you breathe in and going down the *Ren Mai* (front channel) when you breathe out. This is a different style of Qigong and can be done with proper tuition. Some people even like to concentrate on the Dantian, the

Yongquan point (the acupuncture point on the sole of the foot) and so on. These are different methods for people with certain needs. In general, you do not need to do these. The best thing is to follow a qualified Qigong teacher who is healthy.

Some Qigong movements may require certain ways of breathing, such as breathing in as you move up and breathing out when you move down. However, if the movements are in a very long sequence, say in a form like Wild Goose Qigong, the best thing to do is breathe naturally through the nose. Again, different styles of Qigong require different things, and for Healthy Living Gong, the descriptions of the movements will tell you if you need to do any special type of breathing.

If you are unsure how you should breathe, the best thing to do is breathe naturally. There is no harm in this as it is natural and your body will tell you what is best. Ultimately, this way will allow your body to become part of the universe. All will settle into its own rhythm and position without any restrictions.

Qigong is a method that allows your body to go back to nature and become part of it. If you can become one with nature, between heaven and earth, then you will have achieved a high level of Qigong.

How Palms and Face Relate to Health

ONCE I WAS SITTING in the park having tea with my Qigong teacher, Grandmaster Yang Meijun. She pointed to a man walking past and said, 'He has lung problems.' And then she pointed to another person. It was an old man walking past with his head dropped. She said, shaking her head, 'He does not have long to live. All his kidney Qi is gone.' I was impressed by this and wondered how she knew these things.

Later she told me it was from observing the colour of their faces. These are not just the obvious colours that all of us can see, such as bright red cheeks, but something subtler: the colour of the Qi, which reflects the health of the internal organs. These colours relate back to the Five Element theory, each element has a colour that can be observed in the complexion.

I then understood why she had said the man had a lung problem. It was because his face was the white colour of old rice, not a shiny, healthy white. In the five element theory white colour relates to the lungs, so it showed he had breathing problems. The overall texture and quality of the skin also shows how healthy the lungs are. Regarding the second man, whom she said would die soon, his face was black in the area representing the kidneys. If it had been just a little bit dark, my teacher said that maybe he would only have an accident, but because his face was very dark, almost black, she knew that this was a bad sign for the condition of the kidneys. She knew he would not have long to live.

The colour of health

Through my Qigong practise, I understand this, and I also use this method to help diagnose patients. Of course, we often use this skill without even knowing it. If you pet a cat or dog, you can tell their health by the texture and feel of their coat. It is the same with a plant or a tree. If a plant is not healthy, its leaves will change from bright green to yellow. If the condition worsens, the leaf will become dry and brown and soon fall. If the problem is not fixed, the roots will also be affected and the plant will die. If a leaf from a tree is soft and supple and green, then you can tell the tree is in good health. However, if it is dry or has some spots, you know there is a problem somewhere.

It is no different for humans. If you look at our face and palms, you can see all health conditions there. If you have a heart problem, your face will have a deep, even purplish-red colour and be swollen. This red should not be confused with a healthy red, but rather a red that will not go away. There may even be spots or dark veins. It will be the same for the palms. They will have a dark red hue to them. If you have a liver problem, your face will be a sallow yellow or greenish colour, and your palms will be the same. This means there is a problem with the blood circulation resulting from the liver problem.

Today, people like to have plastic surgery and use make-up to try to avoid showing facial signs of ageing or poor health. However, you cannot hide the spirit of the eyes, the colour of the palms and the texture of the skin on the hands. So the state of your health will show more or less on certain parts of your body.

Many people do not understand how to stay healthy. In essence, good health is based on the condition of your internal organs, so if you have a healthy heart, lungs, liver, spleen and kidneys, your skin will glow and your hair will have enough oil. Your eyes will be bright and your face will still look young, even though it may have some lines. No make-up or plastic surgery can replace or copy this. All health conditions start from the inside out.

Because of the Qigong way of looking at things, I have a different concept of beauty. Just because you are young, it does not mean you look good and just because you are old, it does not mean you look bad.

The beauty of health is for all ages. Beauty is not about certain kinds of features or a certain colour of hair or eyes. It is about health shining through. This is because when the channels are open and the internal organs healthy, the eyes will be bright and have good spirit. The skin will be soft and have enough oil naturally. When you are healthy, you will naturally look good and will also attract people who are healthy.

Have you ever noticed that when you practise Qigong you end up meeting similar people? Maybe they practise yoga or Tai Chi, but they have similar interests. People with a good heart who are healthy and have compassion will naturally join together. On the other hand, if you like to take advantage of people, gamble, gossip and put down others, then these will be the kind of people who will come to you. What you are is what you attract.

However, that does not mean to say people cannot change. Practising Qigong will definitely make you healthy and help your heart to change and bring you luck. This is because when you are healthy, you have good energy. When you have good energy, you will attract more positive things. If you are always sad or complaining, do you think that many people will like to be around you? Only the kind of people who have this kind of attitude will want to befriend you.

However, when you are healthy, you will feel good and it is easy to be positive and happy. Lots of people will like to be around you and more good opportunities will open up for you. Just think about a baby when it smiles at you. Can you stop yourself from smiling back?

Healthy people have good luck because when you are healthy, the internal organs and energy in the body is balanced and the mind is clear. When your mind is clear, your judgement will also be clear. So you will not easily be affected by tricky people or someone who is not sincere. You will automatically stay away from those people and know how to develop your life properly. By practising Qigong every day, you will get healthy and the more healthy you are, the more luck you will have.

9

Importance of Correct Posture

WHEN I WAS LITTLE, my father forced my brothers and sister and I to sit straight, walk straight and stand straight. At that time, I did not understand why he was so strict about this. I remember that one time I was supporting my head on my hand and leaning to one side to do my homework. My father came up and shouted at me, 'Sit properly!'

Because of this, I grew up with good posture and now I appreciate what he taught me. Yet while I was growing up I thought that this was just part of Chinese culture, not thinking about it in terms of health. Correct posture is, in fact, part of Confucian thinking and education which says that good behaviour is based on good posture. This philosophy is over 2,500 years old, almost as old as Qigong.

Good posture means having a good foundation. Today, people are very interested in Feng Shui. If a building has a good foundation, this will give it a good structure for the people living or working there. This is the same as having the right posture. With the right posture, your Qi will flow much better and your internal organs will be in the right position and have a good supply of nutrients and Qi.

So how do we find the right posture? If we start with a standing position first, make sure that the weight of your body is distributed evenly over and between both feet. We should not put the weight on one leg or the other too often, otherwise you will develop one side of the organs to be stronger than the other, like kidneys or lungs.

For the Chinese, finding the correct posture is very easy. We use the acupuncture point at the top of the head, called Baihui, and then we align this with the point directly between the legs, called Huiyin (see page 58). This puts the skeleton in the right position. Otherwise, if we rely too much on external body points for correct posture, we may find that because everyone has different proportions and levels of under-standing, then our posture alignment may not be quite right.

When the posture is right, Qi will flow without any blockages along the channels. In this way, the internal organs will get the maximum supply of Qi and you will not feel tired. When you have correct posture, your breathing and body will be in harmony and your mind will be more clear.

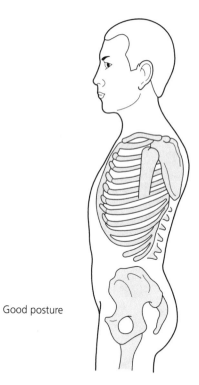

Good posture

Keeping up appearances

In the West, people are more concerned about their appearance, such as having a good figure or nice muscles. However, the more they are con-cerned with trying to tone or build up the external body, then the more it can affect the joints and muscles and also the health of the internal organs. If your joints are stiff, it is very easy to develop arthritis later in life and have aching and spasms in the muscles.

Good posture will allow your Qi to flow without stiffness in your muscles and all your joints will have the relaxation and flexibility to move in all kinds of ways. Today, the most common blockage is in the neck. This will affect the energy going to the brain and also to the eyes, ears, nose and even the teeth. It can even affect your taste. We can see people who have neck problems through their poor posture or dropped heads.

Another very common blockage is the lower back, in the area of the Mingmen point. This can affect the young as well as the old. We move less and less today, using cars instead of walking, using our brain instead of muscles. This can affect the kidneys and liver, and can cause prostate cancer, diabetes and digestive problems as well.

Only you can improve your posture. To do this, you need to be aware of your back all the time. You also need to be aware of your shoulders and make sure they are relaxed and not tense. Be aware of your head, and make sure it is not dropped or leaning forward. Try and use both sides of the body as equally as possible, not just using your right hand but your left. This is not only good for helping to balance your body but also your brain. If you always have good posture, you may even be giving yourself an extra 10 or 20 years of healthy living.

Acupuncture Points

IN BOTH TRADITIONAL Chinese Medicine and Qigong, we use a variety of acupuncture points. Acupuncture points are like doors and windows where Qi enters and is released from the body. These points are located on the various channels in the body.

Our body is like house, so just like in a house, some windows will be small and some will be big, letting in more light. Doorways will let people come and go from the house easily, otherwise no one can leave and no one can come to visit. It is the same for the acupuncture points. Some points are very powerful and will let a lot of Qi go into the body when stimulated. It is these major points that we will use in our Qigong practise.

Some people will refer to these points by numbers but actually you should try to remember their names and what the names mean. This will tell you the essence of the kind of energy that is generated by these points. Below are the points you will use in your practise of Healthy Living Gong and also in meditation. These points are very common and will be used in many of the Qigong forms that I teach.

BAIHUI

Baihui means Sky Door and is on the Du Channel. The Du Channel runs from between the Huiyin point between the legs and up the spine through the Baihui point and down to the upper lip. When the Baihui point is open, then the mind will be clear and calm. It will also help to open our intuition potential. We use this point to help us to find the right posture along with the Huiyin point.

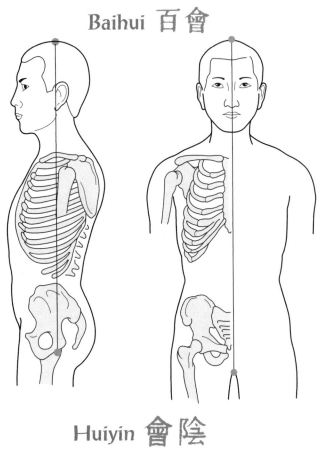

Baihui 百會

Huiyin 會陰

LAOGONG

Laogong means Laboured Place and is on the Pericardium Channel. The Pericardium Channel runs from the middle fingers, up the inside of the arm to the chest. When you close your fingers, the point where the tip of the middle finger touches the palm is the Laogong point. However, when you do more Qigong practise, you will find that you feel heat and sensation not just on this point but in the centre of the whole palm. That is why it is often used for Qi transmission in healing. When you are cold, if you close the palm, you can help retain the heat in your body as this also closes the Laogong point. It is also good for clearing bad smells in the mouth and calming the mind. We use the Laogong points in *Collecting Qi to the Dantian*.

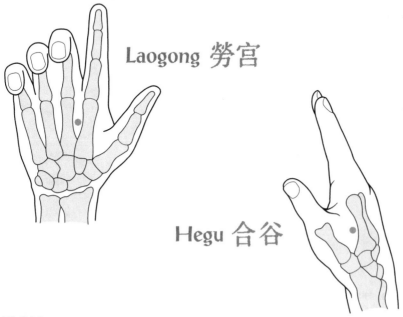

Laogong 勞宮

Hegu 合谷

HEGU

Hegu means Connected Valley and is on the Large Intestine Channel. The Large Intestine Channel runs from the first finger on the outside of the arm, over the shoulder and up to the side of the nose. The Hegu point is located in the valley between the thumb and forefinger. Treating this point helps with headache, toothache and is also good for the common cold. It releases heat from the lungs and liver and is good for blood and Qi circulation. We use the Hegu point in *Separating the Fog to Look for the Clouds* and *Jade Ladder Climbing to the Sky*.

HUANTIAO

Huantiao means Circular Jump and is on the Gall Bladder Channel. The Gall Bladder Channel runs from the head, down the side of the body and legs to the fourth toe. The Huantiao point is located on the sides of the buttocks. This point is a very important Qi point. If Qi is blocked from going through this point, then it will cause hip problems and weakness in the lower body. Because this point is very sensitive, we usually stimulate it only by having another acupuncture point facing it and transmitting Qi to this area. For instance, we use this method in *Jade Ladder Climbing to the Sky*.

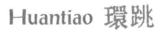

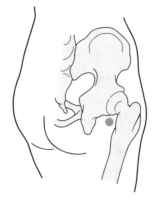

HUIYIN

Huiyin means Yin Energy Meeting Point. This point is located on the Ren Channel directly between the legs. The Ren Channel runs from the Huiyin point up to the lower lip. Treating this point helps with regulating menstruation and strengthening the kidneys. This point can also clear away heat and so help constipation. We often use this point in relation to the Baihui point to help us align our posture. When we have the right body posture, this will allow for the proper flow of Qi through the channels and body.

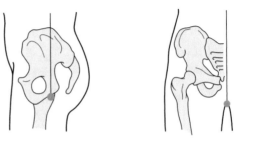

NEIGUAN

Neiguan means Inner Pass and is located on the Pericardium Channel which is a Yin channel. This point is located on the inside of the wrist and treating it helps with heart problems, stomach pain and nervousness. We use the Neiguan points in the movement *Separating the Fog to Look for the Clouds*.

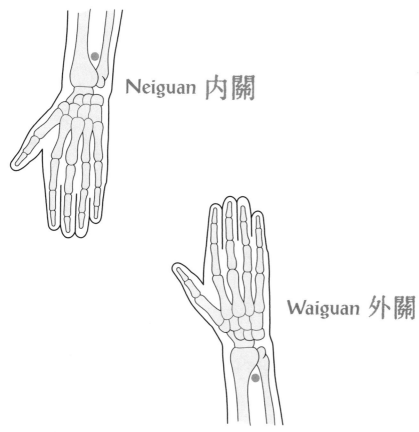

Neiguan 内關

Waiguan 外關

WAIGUAN

Waiguan means Outer Pass and is located on the Sanjiao Channel which is a Yang channel. The Sanjiao Channel runs from the third finger up the shoulder and around the ear to the temple. The Waiquan point is located on the outside of the wrist and treating it helps ringing in the ears, deafness as well as shoulder and arm problems. We use the Waiguan points in the movement *Separating the Fog to Look for the Clouds*.

QUCHI

Quchi means Bending Pond and is on the Large Intestine Channel. This point is located on the edge of the outer crease of the elbow when bent. Treating this point helps joint pain and paralysis in the arms, skin disorders with heat and dizziness. We use this point in the movement *Child Swinging*.

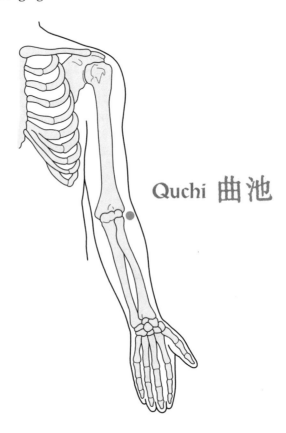

Quchi 曲池

WEIZHONG

Weizhong means Artery Centre and is located on the Urinary Bladder Channel, which runs from the back of the head and down the back of the legs to the small toe. This point is located in the middle of the crease at the back of the knees. Treating it helps with knee problems, swollen legs and arthritis. We use the Weizhong point in the movement *Catching Fish by the Side of the Lake*.

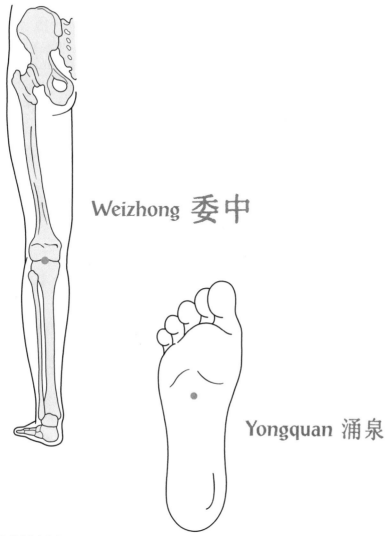

Weizhong 委中

Yongquan 涌泉

YONGQUAN

Yongquan means Pouring Spring and is located on the Kidney Channel which runs from the chest to the soles of the feet. The Yongquan point is located on the soles, just below the balls of the feet. The point is used many times in the Kunlun Dayan System of Qigong and treating it helps to release negative energy from the body. When massaged, it is good for fever and will stimulate the liver and kidneys. We use the Yongquan point in helping us to align our posture while in the low stance of the Ma Bo meditation.

REN CHANNEL

The **Ren Channel** runs from between the legs to the lower lip. It is also called the Conception Channel and it relates to the reproductive organs in the body. When the Qi flows smoothly in this channel, then menstruation will be regular and the reproductive organs will function properly.

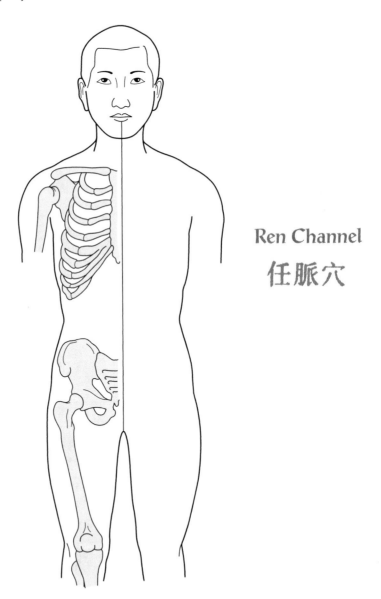

Ren Channel

任脈穴

LOWER, MIDDLE AND UPPER DANTIAN

The **Lower Dantian** is located below the navel and is the area where Qi is stored. It is an area rather than an actual acupuncture point. The more you practise Qigong and the more Qi you store here, then the stronger this area will feel to the touch. You will also have a lot of energy and feel good when the Lower Dantian is full. This area relates to the kidneys and sexual function.

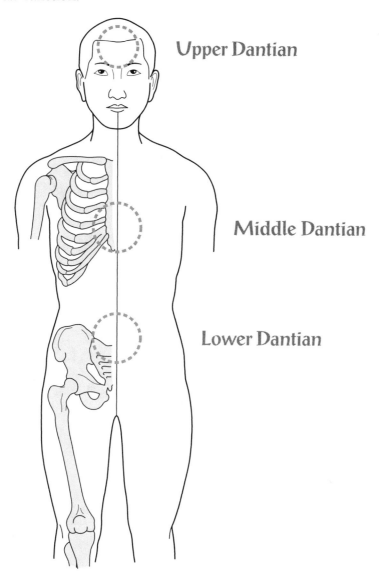

Upper Dantian

Middle Dantian

Lower Dantian

The **Middle Dantian** is located at the middle chest and will store the overflow of Qi from the Lower Dantian as it is converted from Jing (sexual energy) to pure Qi. This area relates to the lungs and breathing.

The **Upper Dantian** is often referred to as the Sky Eye. This area is related to the brain and intuition, seeing colours and receiving messages mentally. When pure Qi rises, it becomes Shen (spiritual) energy. The more Qigong you practise and the more Qi you can store, then this area will start to develop and you will find yourself able to see things more clearly with a calm and unemotional mind.

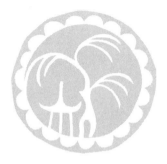

11

Exercises

SOMETIMES WE MAY think we are healthy, but we are really not. For instance, if you think your Qi is strong, try standing in a relaxed posture, with knees slightly bent for ten minutes. If you feel tired after only a few minutes, then it means your bones are weak, and it also means your Qi is weak. When we do Qigong, we strengthen the body from the inside out. We make our heart, lungs, spleen, kidneys and liver strong by gathering fresh Qi to feed them.

When your body is full of Qi, it is stored in the marrow in the bones and stays there like a reserve for when the body needs it. Someone who has good Qi is like a strong, healthy tree. As the tree trunk becomes thicker, the tree gets stronger. You cannot have beautiful, shiny leaves but a weak trunk. The trunk is like our bones, the leaves are like our skin and hair, and the roots are like our legs. Everything is connected and nothing is individual and separate.

So you should not forget that to be healthy, your Qigong exercises must include relaxation, good coordination and also fitness. This will make not only your body healthy, but also your thinking, and this is very important. The following exercises cover both body and mind, and meditation is covered in Chapter 12.

Healthy Living Gong Exercises

Notes on practising

SEQUENCE

In the beginning, you should learn and practise each movement in order, and practise this way for a few weeks. The best method is to read all of the movement descriptions and match them to the pictures. Then fully read about the breathing, concentration, background and benefits as this will help you understand more about using the right emphasis for the movement. Once you have done this, you are ready to try the movement.

My suggestion is to not learn more than three movements in one session, doing a minimum of ten or twelve repetitions of each. However, most people like the movements so much that they enjoy doing more. You should take your time to practise the new movements for a few days, until you can do them without referring back to the book. This will help you to understand the movements and to get the right energy and gain the most health benefit. If you try to rush and learn the movements all at once, you may confuse yourself.

I would suggest that in the beginning you practise the movements in the order presented. When you practise all of the movements in order, this will help build up a proper foundation, going from proper posture, relaxation, flexibility and coordination. When you are familiar with all the exercises, you can choose your favourites or the individual ones which will help with a particular health problem. (See Appendix I for a chart of illnesses/health problems matched with the appropriate exercise.)

WHEN TO PRACTISE

If you can set aside the same time every day to do your practise, such as morning, afternoon or evening, this will help you to develop a routine. It is human nature to be a bit lazy, but if you want to have good results, you should still try to practise, even for just five or ten minutes a day.

You will find that even after a few minutes you will start to enjoy yourself and feel better.

FINISHING

When you have completely finished with all of your exercises and are ready to do your Qigong meditation, you should then do a finishing movement called Shou Gong. This movement is described in Chapter 12, in the section on meditation (page 116). Shou Gong is only done when you are finished with your practise, not between each movement. Otherwise it will interrupt the energy. Having a good ending is even more important than having a good beginning, because every ending is just a new beginning.

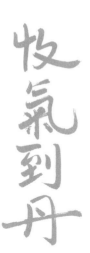

Collecting Qi to the Dantian

GOOD FOR • Dantian • Circulation • Insomnia

ACUPUNCTURE POINTS Laogong (see page 58) and Ren Channel (see page 64)

1 Stand with your feet shoulder-width apart, knees slightly bent and your back straight.

2 Shift your weight slightly to the left and start to raise your left hand to the side of the body.

3 Continue to bring the left arm upwards to the Sky Eye (see page 66) and at the same time move the body back to the centre in the starting position.

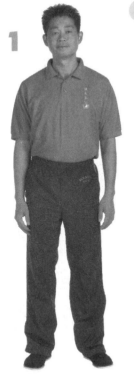

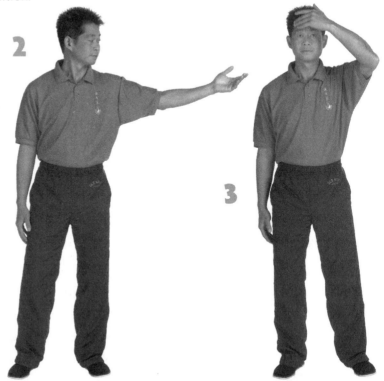

4 When the left hand reaches the Sky Eye, start to shift the body to the right and lift the right arm out to the side of the body. Both hands will move continuously in a cycling motion, so when one hand is at mid-chest, the other hand will be out to the side of the body. The body follows whichever hand starts to lift upwards.

5 Let the right hand continue upwards to the Sky Eye and the left hand sink to the Lower Dantian.

Keep repeating the above movements and cycling your arms to the left and right. As one hand raises, the other hand should be moving downwards, both balanced.

6 To finish the movement, let both hands sink one at a time back to the Lower Dantian and then straighten the legs.

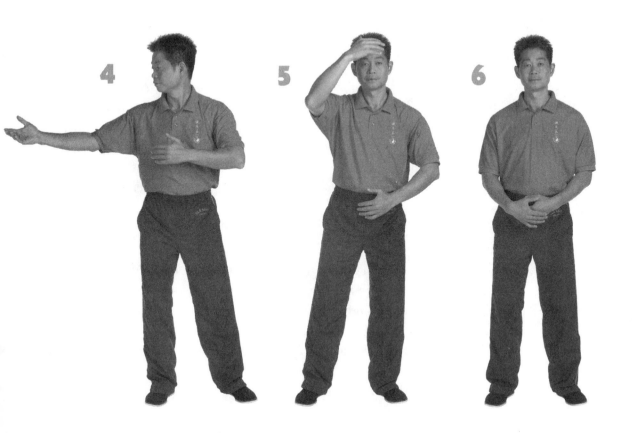

BREATHING

As one hand raises, breathe in and when the other hand raises on the other side of the body, breathe out. Breathe naturally through your nose. When doing this exercise, you do not need to think about your breathing too much. It is more important to be relaxed.

CONCENTRATION

Make sure that your eyes follow the rising hand. Both hands should move continuously, balancing themselves between top and bottom. If one hand is at the Sky Eye, then the other should be at the Lower Dantian. In this way your hands are always opposite and balanced. If you find that you cannot keep the balance between the hands as you move them simultaneously, then it means that one side of your brain is stronger than the other or that you are doing the movements too quickly, not connecting with your breathing.

BACKGROUND/HISTORY

If you have done *Green Sea Swimming Dragon Gong* (a form which is part of the Qigong syllabus that I teach), you will recognise that this Healthy Living Gong movement comes from the Swimming Dragon movement, *Fostering Qi in a Circle*. However, unlike *Fostering Qi in a Circle*, we do not walk but stay in one place. However, at the end of these exercises there is a walking exercise. It is based on *Collecting Qi to the Dantian*.

HEALTH BENEFITS

This movement is very good for coordination. In the West, looking good externally is the main emphasis for health. Coordination is not considered, even though it actually plays a major role in health. If someone moves clumsily, it means they will be prone to strokes and high blood pressure in the future. The brain plays a great part in our health. We cannot have good health without the brain being able to think clearly and control the movements of the body. For example, if you want to move your left arm, but you usually use only the right arm, your left side will be weak. Unless you work to balance both sides of the body equally, your weak side will not work properly when you want to move it, so the right side of the brain will develop a problem. This is because the energy in the body crosses over, the left brain controlling the right side of the body, etc.

When we let our emotions get too strong, like losing our temper or doing something that uses more energy than we have, like lifting something very heavy, then the weak side of the brain will be affected. This is because there is not enough blood and Qi to balance the brain and body together. The brain will not be able to cope with the stimulus and it might lead to a stroke. So good coordination is very important as it avoids imbalances in the brain and keeps us healthy and younger.

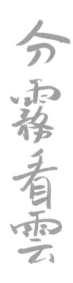

Separating the Fog to Look for the Clouds

> **GOOD FOR** • Stomach • Digestive system • Breathing
>
> **ACUPUNCTURE POINTS** Neiguan (see page 61), Waiguan (see page 61) and Hegu (see page 59)

1 Stand with your feet shoulder-width apart, knees slightly bent and your back straight. Cross your wrists in front of your Lower Dantian (see page 65), palms facing upwards. Men should place their left hand over the right hand. Ladies should place their right over the left hand. The Neiguan and Waiguan points (see page 61) should be close together.

2 Turn the palms so they are facing downwards.

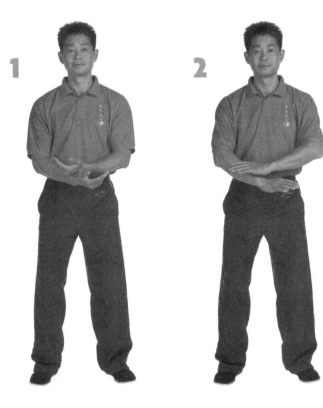

3 Open both hands out to the side of the body, keeping the Hegu points (see page 59) facing each other. As you open the hands, straighten the legs.

4 Turn the palms upwards and simultaneously bring your hands back to the starting position while bending the knees.

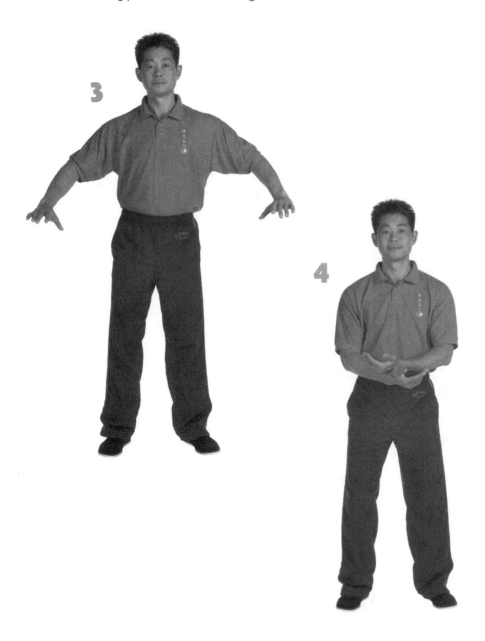

BREATHING

As your hands open to the side of the body, breathe in. As they close, breathe out. Make sure that you breathe naturally through the nose.

CONCENTRATION

It is important to keep the back straight, regardless of separating or closing the hands. Some people may have a tendency to collapse the chest when they close the hands back to the starting position. If you do this, you will affect the lungs and breathing.

When you separate the hands out to the side of the body, the Hegu points should face each other. Keep your elbows bent when you separate the hands, so the arms form a semi-circle. The arms should not be completely straight as this will create tension in the shoulders and back. Make sure that you look forward and do not drop the head. Your mind should lightly think about the Dantian, but do not concentrate on it too hard.

BACKGROUND/HISTORY

This movement is a little like the movement called *Opening and Closing the Dantian*, which is from a set of Qigong exercises that I created in 1993 called Balancing Gong and which can be found in my book, *Qigong for Health & Vitality* (Piatkus). In the Healthy Living Gong movement, *Separating the Fog to Look for the Clouds*, the Hegu points face each other and the arms make a semi-circle out to the sides of the body, not in front of the body. However, in the Balancing Gong movement, *Opening and Closing Dantian*, the hands form a full circle and the Hegu points face the Daimai points just inside the hip bones.

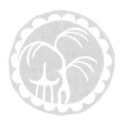

BENEFITS

Separating the Fog to Look for the Clouds is good for the stomach and intestines, urinary bladder, sexual organs and menstrual problems. As well as those mentioned above, this movement is good for the lower part of the body, from the chest down to the the area between the legs. It is good for the 'Lower Warmer' (Lower Jiao), meaning the stomach, liver, large intestine, small intestine, urinary bladder and reproductive organs.

It can help with illnesses such as constipation and problems with the reproductive organs. This movement is especially good for women, but it will help men as well.

湖
畔
捉
魚

Catching Fish by the Side of the Lake

GOOD FOR • Low blood pressure • Circulation • Headache

ACUPUNCTURE POINT Weizhong (see page 62)

1 Bend forward, keeping both legs straight. Let arms relax to the sides.

2 Move the right hand towards the right leg in a clockwise direction and touch the Weizhong point which is on the back of the knee (see page 62). When moving the hand, keep the palm facing the ground.

3 After your right hand touches the Weizhong point, move the left hand towards the front of the right knee.

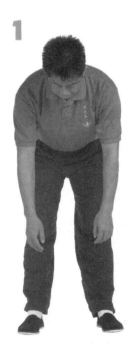

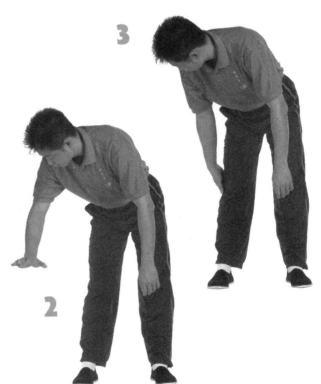

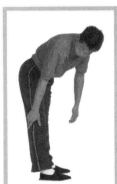

4 Circle the left arm in an anticlockwise direction to touch the Weizhong point on the left leg.

5 As your left hand touches the left Weizhong point, start to move the right hand towards the left knee and then move outwards in a clockwise circle to the right Weizhong point.

6 Keep repeating, making the movement continuous. As one hand is coming to the back, the other is pushing out. Each time you circle your hand, it should come to rest at the Weizhong point.

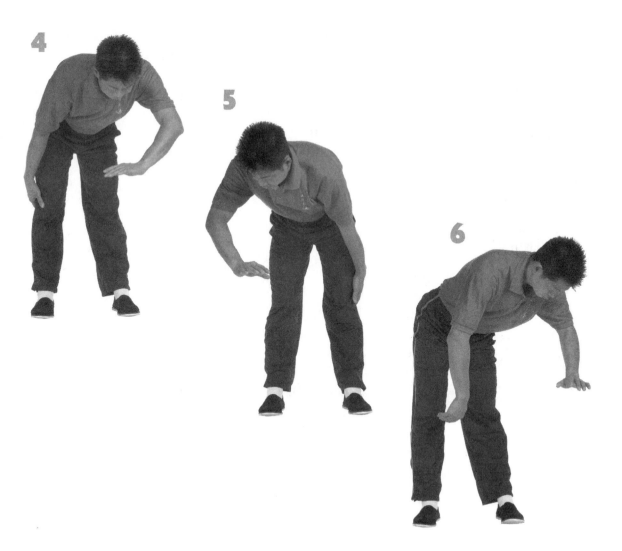

BREATHING

When one hand is making a circle, breathe in and when the other makes its circle, breathe out. Breathe naturally and do not think about it.

CONCENTRATION

Concentrate and look at the hand that is going out, not the one coming to touch the Weizhong point. Make sure that you keep the knees straight and only let the upper body move from side to side. Actually, the circling of the arms is mostly due to the movement from the waist as it gently moves from side to side. Do not drop the head too much but keep it slightly lifted and looking at the hands as they move. If you find you are dizzy at all when doing this movement, then make sure you are not bending over too far or dropping the head below the waist. If you still feel dizzy after correcting these points, then raise the upper body a little higher, but do not be afraid and try to avoid the movement. Otherwise, you will never fix the problem and it may even get worse.

BENEFITS

This is good for the lower back, waist and the kidneys. Your back is very important for the flow of your energy. If your back is stiff, then it means you are getting old. You must fix this by making the back more flexible again. If you allow your back to become stiff, then all your movements will become stiff. With a stiff back, you can develop back pain and kidney problems. You will also have problems with your shoulders and neck. So the back is very important for all the joints in the body.

The waist is like the steering wheel of a car. If you have a problem with the steering wheel, then you can easily have an accident. Bending forwards is good for easing headaches and for people with low blood pressure. When the head does not get enough blood and Qi flowing to it, this will cause headaches, even migraines. This is the same as having low blood pressure. If the circulation is poor, of course we will not have enough blood flowing around the body. This is particularly true for women, as during their period they lose a lot of blood. During this time they can easily have headaches, cold hands and feet and their emotions are also affected.

As we lean forward, this brings the Qi and blood to the upper body. People with high blood pressure may find it difficult to bend forward and people with low blood pressure might find it harder to stretch up with their hands up.

HISTORY/BACKGROUND

This movement does not come from any other exercise that I have been practising. It comes from my childhood when my parents would take our family back to my mother's village, Tong Ha, to visit relatives. There they kept a lot of fish in a pond. When they wanted to eat fish, they would just go out to the pond and catch some. They would only eat very fresh fish, unlike what we eat today, which may have been standing around for a long time. They used a net to catch the fish and would bend over the edge of the pond to get them.

I imagined standing in the pond (which was not so deep) and seeing all the fish swimming around. Then I would bend over and try to catch them with my hand. Of course, I would never catch one, so I could keep doing the movement without hurting any of them.

Having done a lot of standing exercises, I know that bending down is a very useful movement which can keep the back flexible. The Weizhong point belongs to the urinary bladder channel. The urinary bladder is very closely related to the kidneys, like a brother, and so stimulating this point is good for the kidneys as well.

五
爪
金
龍

Golden Dragon Stretches Its Claws

GOOD FOR • Arthritis • Coordination • Finger injury

1 Stand with your left foot forward and your right foot back. All your weight should be on the back leg, which is bent. Your left leg (front leg) should be straight and light. Hold your left hand at around ear level and your right hand by your waist. Both hands should be held like dragons' claws with the fingers slightly rounded and the palm hollowed. The waist should be open, with the upper body turning 45 degrees to the right.

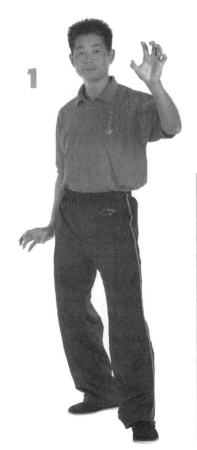
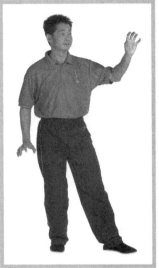

2 Simultaneously shift your weight forward on the left leg and let your arms rotate so your left arm cycles in a circle downwards and your right hand cycles upwards in a circle. Make sure to keep the hands held like dragons' claws.

Repeat, moving your weight forward and backward while cycling the arms as many times as you like.

3 Now, change your feet, so your right foot is forward and your left foot is behind, so that the position is opposite to that used in the beginning. Repeat the same movement again and again until you feel good.

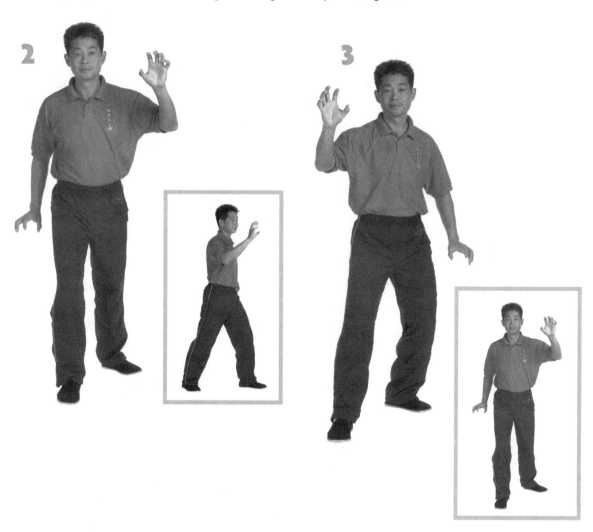

BREATHING

As your body moves forward, breathe out and as the body moves backwards, breathe in. If you cannot manage to coordinate the movement and the breathing, just breathe naturally, as this is also good.

CONCENTRATION

Keep all the joints in your arms and hands bent all the time, particularly the fingers and arms as they move forward. Never fully stretch out the arms so that they are tense or close them up too tight to the body. Keep the same relaxed shape all the time, as though the arms were moving in a circle and as if you are holding a ball in each hand.

The movement should come from the waist and you should look at the hand that is moving forwards. As the body moves forward, the waist should face forward. As the weight shifts backwards on to the back leg, then the waist opens 45 degrees. It is important to keep all your joints relaxed, including the hands. They should not be tense.

Always remember that whichever leg is bent, the opposite hand to this leg should also be the one to cycle forward.

BENEFITS

This exercise is very good for your coordination. Many people think that as long as the movement flows well, it will make them healthy, and so they are not bothered to keep the correct hand position. However, they forget that coordination is also very important. Those with good co-ordination will also have clear minds and will always think about the circumstances they are in. They will think about other people more and will not be so short-sighted. Coordination is not only about developing the muscles, but it is also to do with improving the functioning of the brain.

If you cannot do more than one thing at a time, it means that there is not enough energy going to the brain. When this happens, people can easily feel under stress. When someone can do more than one thing at a time, they can think about the next step or what effect their action will have on the future. This is because they have enough energy going to the brain. If you have more Qi going to the brain, your mind will be clearer and you can cope with whatever happens.

When all the joints are relaxed, this allows the Qi to flow through all the channels. This movement is particularly good for people with arthritis or rheumatism. These problems start because the Qi cannot go through the channels and so all the toxins build up in the joints. However, even if you do not suffer from these problems, this exercise will still be good for your joints and circulation, especially the knees and ankles, shoulders and elbows.

HISTORY/BACKGROUND

Have you ever seen drawings and paintings of Chinese dragons? These differ from those in the West. The Chinese dragon is the symbol of the king or emperor who was the leader of all China. In the past, it was said that no matter who governed the country, this person was a dragon who had come down to earth just for this purpose. So the emperor's clothes would always have a dragon emblem embroidered on them and they would always be yellow. Yellow is the colour of the element earth. In the Five Element theory, Earth is in the middle, so this symbolised that the emperor was like the centre, or stable foundation, of all China.

Chinese dragons could fly without wings and had claws with five fingers. The claws symbolised the Five Elements and all the directions in the world. So a dragon emblem was only allowed to be seen on the emperor's clothes and other personal things. No one else was allowed to use it, otherwise they would be imprisoned or even killed, because the dragon symbolised the emperor, the Son of Heaven, and only the emperor was supposed to have this level of power. Today, though, this is not a problem. I created this movement with the hope that every one of us can be like a Chinese dragon, with strong and flowing energy.

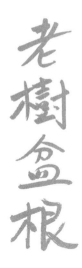

Old Tree with Winding Roots

GOOD FOR • Ground energy • Strengthening legs • Kidneys

ACUPUNCTURE POINTS Neiguan (see page 61) and Waiguan (see page 61)

1 Stand with your weight on your left leg and the knee slightly bent. Place the right foot next to it, heel up, only the toes touching. Cross your wrists in front of your Lower Dantian (see page 65). Men should place the left hand over the right and women, the right over the left. Allow the Neiguan and Waiguan points (see page 61) to connect together in front of the Dantian.

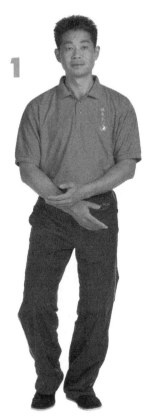

2 Step to the right with your right foot, while keeping both knees bent and the weight even on both legs. As you step, separate the hands so the fingertips lightly touch the liver and spleen on either side of the body. Do not touch with the palms. Make sure the back is straight and the shoulders back and chest open as you open the legs.

3 Step towards the right foot, with the left foot, keeping both knees bent at the same level as before. The left heel should be up and all the weight should be on the right leg. At the same time as you step, bring your hands back to the same position at the Lower Dantian as before.

Repeat the stepping and closing, moving from left to right and right to left.

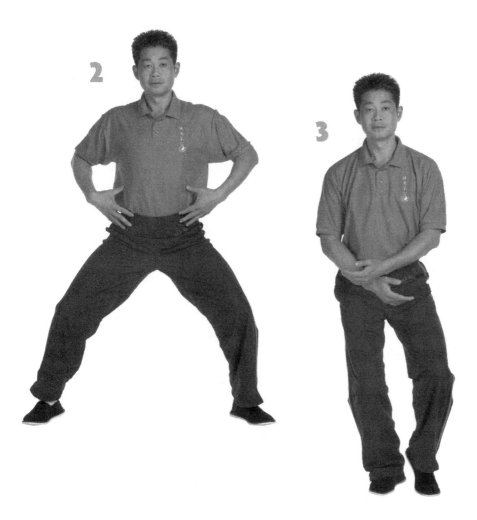

BREATHING

As you step open, breathe in and as you close, breathe out. Do not breathe any other way.

CONCENTRATION

Breathing is very important in this movement. It is a special kind of breathing called 'reverse breathing'. With reverse breathing, when you breathe in, the Dantian will go in and when you breathe out, the Dantian will push out. This is just the opposite of normal or natural breathing. (For more information on breathing, refer to Chapter 7.)

This movement will allow you to gather and also to ground the Qi. When you open, make sure the body stays at the same level as your starting position. Do not let the body move up and down as you open and close. In the beginning, some people may find their legs are quite weak, so when they close the legs together after doing the opening, they will try to straighten the legs. However, if you do this you will lose Qi. Also, when you close the legs, keep the body facing forward. You should not have the body turned to the side.

BENEFITS

This exercise is very good for the lungs. Many people today find that when they try to breathe deeply, it is too difficult to do so through the nose and, instead, they will open their mouth to breathe. This is because their lungs have not been exercised enough. Our lungs are muscles, the same as the leg muscles. If you do not work them, they will become weak. Then, when you need to run or climb stairs or do something a bit strenuous, you will have no energy.

Another benefit of this exercise is that it helps strengthen the legs. A healthy person cannot live without strong legs as legs are the root of our body. It is the same as using a tripod for your camera. If the tripod is too weak to support your camera, what will happen? We all know what the result will be. Strong and balanced legs are very important. This movement also benefits the stomach, spleen and liver so the internal organs will become strong and healthy.

HISTORY

This exercise was inspired by my Chen Taijiquan training, as well as the principle in Chinese culture that legs are the root of our bodies. Chen Taijiquan training is very much about the legs. Strong legs can bring you a lot of energy, make the body warm and the foundation strong.

In Chinese culture, we always hear about the ten generations of the Tang family and twenty generations of the Kong family. In the West we do not hear too much about these sorts of things, because in the West people are educated to make as much money as they can, to be as famous as they can, as these are considered to be marks of success. I do not mean that you should not be rich and famous. There are a lot of good rich and famous people. But today's education does not tell us to respect our parents who cared for us when we were little, when we were too small to feed ourselves or go to the toilet alone.

Nor does it teach people to respect the teachers who taught them so that they could make their living in the future. It is your teacher who taught you how to read and write, and how to respect your boss who pays your wages so you can keep your finances in good order.

All of these are your roots. Of course there are bad teachers, but if everyone was educated to respect their ancestors, their teachers, their family, their employer, there would be less problems in the world today. Just because others show disrespect, it does not mean that we should do the same. If someone else steals, it does not mean you should steal.

The Chinese see their ancestors as their power and their roots. With strong roots, then the tree will be strong and the leaves and the fruit will be good. If you had many generations living together under one roof, this was considered very lucky and must mean that your family had done a lot of good things. Anyone who has many generations in their family is proof that their roots are strong and healthy and that their family tree can grow fruits and flowers.

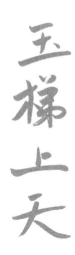

Jade Ladder Climbing to the Sky

> **GOOD FOR** • Coordination • High blood pressure • Chronic fatigue syndrome (ME)
>
> **ACCUPUNCTURE POINTS** Laogong (see page 58) and Huantiao (see page 59)

1 Stand relaxed with your feet together and your arms by the side of your body and the Laogong points facing the Huantiao points.

2 Lift up your left leg so that it is level with your waist, and at the same time, stretch up your left hand above the head so that the palm faces towards the right. As you lift up the arm, straighten the right leg. The Laogong point of your right palm should remain facing the right Huantiao point with the fingers closed in a relaxed position. Keep your eyes looking forwards.

3 Slowly turn your left palm outwards and make a hollow fist. Then slowly lower both your left leg and arm down.

4 As the left leg moves downwards, bend the right leg and let the left foot settle beside the right foot and let the left hand drop down to your side and face the Huantiao point. Pause slightly.

Repeat the movement for the right hand. Continue repeating the movement as many times as you like or until you feel good.

BREATHING

As you lift up your hand and leg, breathe in. As you drop your hand and leg, breathe out.

CONCENTRATION

When you raise up your hand, make sure that you stretch the arm gently upwards, so that it is straight above the head. This will open your

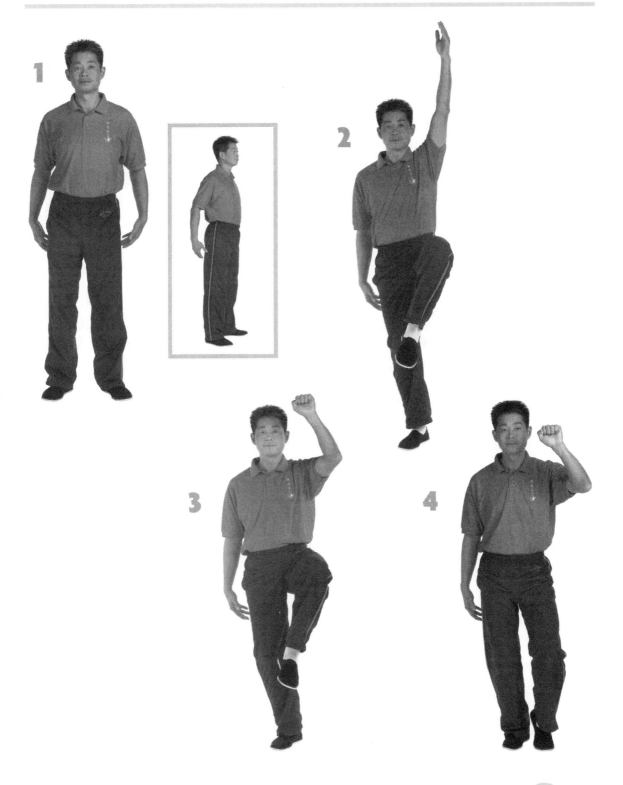

chest and benefit your heart and lungs. Before you drop your hand and leg, pause and balance on one leg for a very short moment before going back to the starting position. Keep the eyes looking forward as you raise and lower the hand. As you lower the hand and leg, make sure that you move slowly in order to control your energy and your weight. As you lower the raised leg, you should also bend the standing leg until you end back up in the starting position with both legs bent slightly. The weight should be on the thighs and back straight. You should also pause slightly before continuing with the movement. Pay attention to the acupuncture points that we use, that is, the Laogong and Huantiao points, because these points are doors for Qi to enter the body.

BENEFITS

Some people find that standing on one leg is not easy. If this is the case, you might be more susceptible to high blood pressure and strokes. When you stand on one leg, you need to relax your mind. If your mind is under stress, it will not have enough energy to function clearly and you will find it hard to concentrate and think. Standing on one leg is not about how strong your muscles are, it is about the balance of Qi in your brain. Just because someone has big muscles, it does not necessarily mean that they can stand on one leg for a long time.

Therefore, this exercise is very good for your brain and for balancing your blood circulation. In order to be able to do this movement properly, the blood must flow along the body properly, instead of relying on big muscles. This is why standing on one leg can prevent strokes and high blood pressure. Another benefit is opening your chest when you reach up. It is very common for us to have poor posture and, without even knowing it, we will close our chests and hunch our shoulders. This is not good for your health and will damage the internal organs. It is like having wrinkles in your clothes. If your clothes are very wrinkled, you will never look neat, tidy and bright. It is the same as wrinkling up your internal organs. In the long run, how can you be healthy?

A deformed posture not only makes you tired. If it continues, it can make you ill and it will affect your brain and thinking. Eventually, you might not be able to get your good posture back. The key to good posture is to straighten your back. *Jade Ladder Climbing to the Sky* is very good for this. When the posture is correct, it will also open the Qihu points which is good for our breathing. (If you place your four fingers under your armpit of the opposite arm and close your arm on your hand, your thumb will rest on your Qihu point on your chest.) Lastly, opening the chest and looking forward with the eyes will help you to stop dropping your head and deforming your posture.

HISTORY

The origin of this movement is quite obvious as it looks as if you are climbing a ladder. I called it 'Jade Ladder' as this is a very Chinese name. The idea behind it is that we need to exercise while standing on one leg. This will test our balance. I find that today, many Qigong exercises are done standing on both legs and so do not challenge the body enough. If you do not try and stand on one leg, how can you say you are healthy? You might be able to stand on both legs for half an hour, but cannot maintain a good balance and stand for even 10 seconds on one leg. If this is the case, then you have a problem with brain coordination and cannot claim to be really healthy.

A good concept of health is that you can do things the majority of other people can do, such as balancing on one leg, bending over without feeling dizzy, sitting on the floor for half an hour without feeling pain when you get up, walking up the stairs without puffing and panting at the top, running and jumping a certain distance and height without a problem. If you can, then you are probably quite healthy.

If you find there is something that most people can do that you cannot, the first thing to do is to face it and not hide or try to avoid it. Do not feel embarrassed. When you face the problem, the mind will relax when you start to change and cope with the problem and so you will get healthier. Then you need to work on it with the physical body. Each time you overcome certain movements and difficulties of thinking, your health will get better. Gradually, you will become a very healthy person.

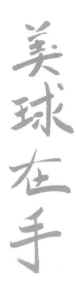

Holding the Beautiful Ball

GOOD FOR • Cold • Asthma • Bronchitis

ACUPUNCTURE POINT Laogong (see page 58)

1 Stand still with your feet shoulder-width apart and knees slightly bent. Hold the hands slightly wider than the body at the level of the Lower Dantian (see page 65) as if holding a large ball between them. The Laogong points should face each other.

2 Straighten the legs and lift up the arms upwards to the Middle Dantian (see page 66).

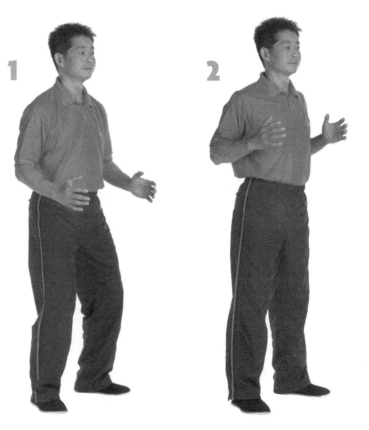

3 Rotate the arms forward, keeping the Laogong points facing each other.

4 Then lower your arms to the Lower Dantian level while still holding the Qi ball. When you lower the arms, bend the knees slightly.

5 Pull back your hands to the starting position, keeping the knees bent and repeat the cycle. You should have made a circle with your hands, firstly going upwards, then forwards and down and then back to the starting position. When moving the hands, make sure the movement is smooth and the cycling uninterupted.

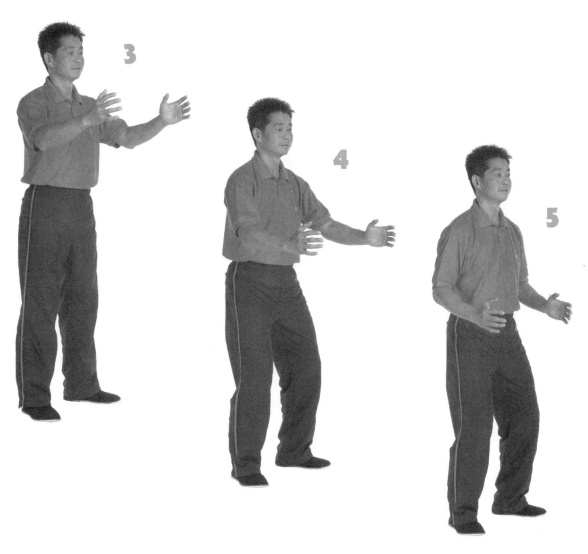

BREATHING

As you lift up your hands to the chest, breathe in. As you lower your hands and bend your knees, breathe out.

CONCENTRATION

Make sure to open your chest when you lift up your hands as this will benefit your lungs and heart. Keep your hands apart on either side of the body with Laogong point facing Laogong point. If you hold your hands closer, it will make the shoulders tense when you lift your arms upwards.

BENEFITS

This is the simplest exercise of all we have done so far. Although it is simple, it is very good for our health condition, particularly our lungs and heart. In fact, simple exercises do not mean the benefit they offer is small, and complicated exercises do not mean that they are the best for health. It all depends on how the exercise works for the internal body. Today, I see so many people who have poor posture. They either drop the head, tense up the shoulders, close their chest or bend over in a crooked posture. These habits all deform our bodies and squeeze up our internal organs. As a result, our internal organs will not have enough energy. They will also create blockages which will make us unhealthy and affect our emotions.

A good Traditional Chinese Medicine (TCM) doctor will look at the appearance and mannerisms of a person and then make a diagnosis of their problem. This is called observation and is one of four methods of diagnosis in TCM. The others are smelling (each organ has its own smell in both health and sickness), asking and testing the pulse. However, even as you walk into the room, a good doctor will already be able to see your problem.

A healthy person will have good spirit and good posture, standing upright and looking forward. Facial colour will be good, and their eyes will show good spirit. Their voice will be clear and not weak. An unhealthy person will have poor posture, low energy, loss of eye spirit and a weak voice.

In this way, TCM is similar to Chinese palm and face telling. A face and palm reader will not just look at your face and palm. They will also look at your attitude to prove their predictions correct. For instance, a person may have a lucky face, but if their posture is crooked and their breathing poor, then it means their luck will not last. So you have to consider the whole attitude of a person. I remember my father saying to me, 'Head dropped and no eye spirit, then even if there is money on the street, you will miss it.' This means if someone's energy is gone, then their body will start to be bent and their overall health and luck will also go down. So having strong and healthy lungs and heart is very important for your luck.

HISTORY/BACKGROUND

I met my first Taijiquan teacher almost 20 years ago. His name was Fung Man Yiu. Once we were talking about people using a Taiji ruler to practise Qigong. A Taiji ruler is a piece of wood with rounded ends which are held against the Laogong points while holding it between the palms and rotating it in a circle. The exercise is similar to *Holding the Beautiful Ball*. People say that when you practise with the Taiji ruler, all the negative energy will go to the ruler.

Therefore, you should not let other people use your ruler or use theirs as you might pass on or take on other people's negative energy. This is very true. Any tool or weapon you use will have your energy stored in it. Either you will have good or bad energy, and that energy will connect together with the weapon. If you are not well, anything you regularly use will have your negative energy. However, if you are healthy, then whatever you use will have your good energy. So if someone uses your things when you are healthy, they will benefit.

Personally, I prefer to practise without the ruler as I feel the energy is even stronger, and you can also practise any time you want. When it comes to lifting up your hands, it is easier to do without the ruler, which can cause the shoulders to be tense and the chest not to open enough. Without the ruler, the movement will flow more freely and open the chest more.

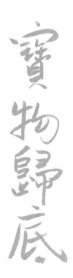

Looking for Treasure at the Bottom of the Chest

GOOD FOR • Backache • Kidneys • Heart

1 Stand straight with elbows loosely bent and arms open to the sides of the body.

2 Lean forwards from the waist and bring the hands to the Lower Dantian (see page 65), so that palms are facing this area. Make sure elbows are rounded and open, not close against the body.

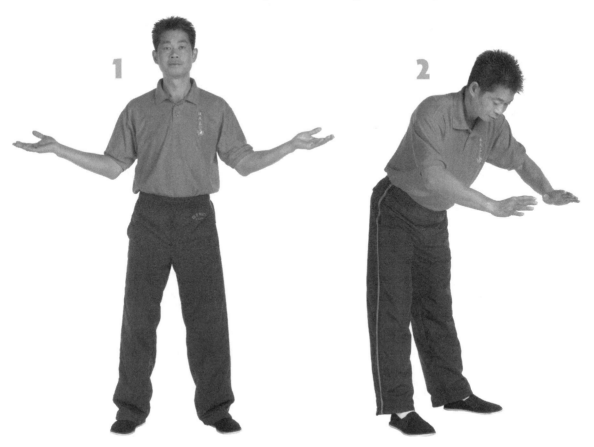

3 Touch the thumbs to the middle fingers.

4 Lean back with knees slightly bent and open the arms to the sides of the body. Look upwards slightly, keeping the elbows and wrists relaxed and fingers touching.

Repeat the movement as you lean forward again and again.

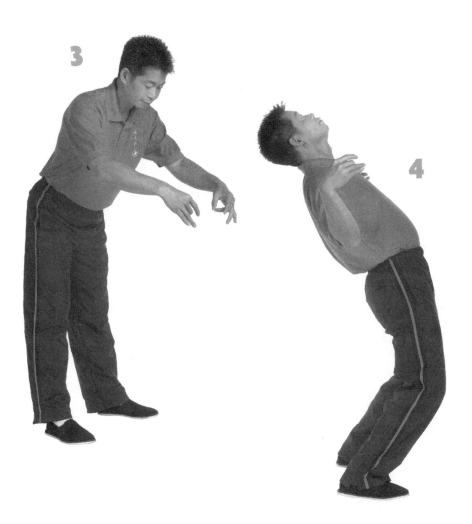

BREATHING

When you bend forward, breathe out and as you lean backward, breathe in.

CONCENTRATION

When you are bent over at the waist, make sure the knees are straight and that the hands are held at the Lower Dantian level. In this position, the elbows should be out and the middle finger and thumb tips touching, as this precedes leaning backwards. When you lean backwards, look upwards slightly. The knees will be slightly bent and the elbows will be held closer to the body with the palms open in this position. When you lean forwards, open the palms so that you gather energy instead of connecting the fingers together.

This movement is quite gentle. The arms do not open too much, and the hands should not be higher than the Middle Dantian (middle chest height) (see page 66) when open to the sides.

BENEFITS

The Lower Dantian and kidneys are two of the most important parts of the body and relate to Qi. These areas store energy in order for us to live longer and for when we need it. Maintaining the kidneys and strengthening the Dantian are very important for health. By doing *Looking for Treasure at the Bottom of the Chest*, we work for the kidneys and the back when we lean backwards. When we touch our fingers together, the middle finger relates to the heart and the thumb relates to the spleen. So when we connect them together, we stimulate these two organs to make the Qi stronger.

Also, in the Five Element theory, the heart relates to the element fire and kidneys relate to water. Fire and water coming together creates a lot of energy, like Yin and Yang. Everything we relate to has opposite sides, like Yin and Yang, fire and water.

For example, when you make bread, you need both water and fire. When you cook, you need water and fire. When you do your laundry, you need water to wash the clothes and heat to dry the clothing. This is how we make things develop. When we lean forward in the movement and touch the fingers, we stimulate the heart fire and when we lean back, we stimulate the kidney water.

HISTORY/BACKGROUND

Looking for Treasure at the Bottom of the Chest is a Chinese metaphor meaning that all the best things are always at the bottom or at the end. In the old times, when you went to the market to buy something, usually the best part would be kept in the back or hidden at the bottom. First, the sellers would only show you the ordinary one. In most Chinese households, families like to keep valuable things hidden underneath the bed or hidden in the bottom of a case or chest.

So usually, we will say if you are the last one to be chosen for a job, you are the most lucky one. That is what we mean when we say *Looking for Treasure at the Bottom of the Chest*. I used this phrase to relate to this movement as it looks like we are looking for something at the bottom of the chest and at the same time to connect with the kidney movement. This is because the kidneys are one of our most precious internal organs.

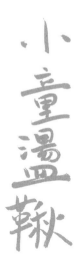

Child Swinging

GOOD FOR • Arthritis • Tennis elbow • Circulation
ACUPUNCTURE POINT Quchi (see page 62)

1 Bend your left knee and lean body sideways and fully extend the left arm with palm facing backward. The right arm should be bent with the fingers touching the left Quchi point (see page 62), which is just on the crease of the elbow when it is bent.

2 Move the body back towards the centre while simultaneously closing the left hand over the right arm so the left fingers are now touching the right Quchi point. The right hand will still be briefly touching the left

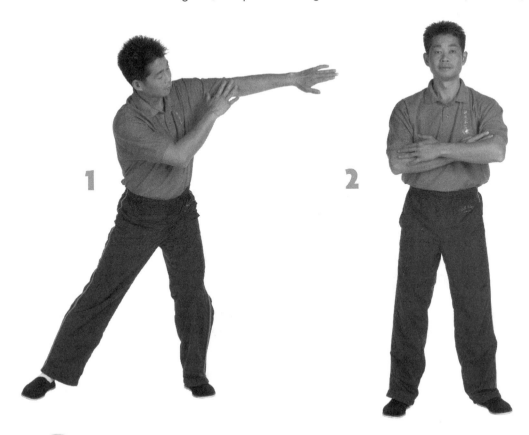

Quchi point before commencing the next movement. The legs should be straight and even.

3 Bend the right knee and lean the body to the right side. Simultaneously swing the right arm downwards and then upwards again in an arc. The right palm should be facing backwards and left fingers still touching the Quchi point.

4 Swing the body back to the centre and this time fold the right hand over the left arm so that the right fingers are now touching the left Quchi point.

Repeat the exercise on both sides until you feel happy and healthy. When you are ready to finish, fold the left arm over the right arm and straighten both legs and stand straight.

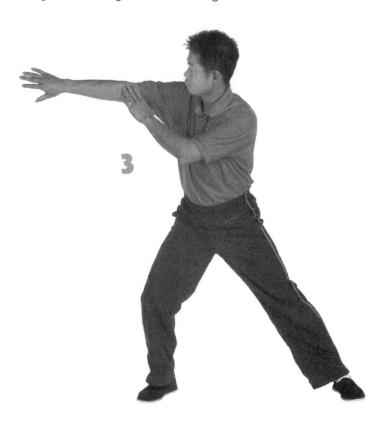

BREATHING

For breathing, you breathe in on one side and breathe out on the other. Otherwise, just breathe naturally and do not think about it.

CONCENTRATION

When you do the exercise, do not concentrate on the hands. You should concentrate on the waist. As you shift the weight to one side, make sure the movement comes from the waist. The hands are just for connecting the energy. When you swing your arms, the fingertips of one hand should touch the Quchi point of the opposite hand.

BENEFITS

Today, so many people work on the computer and use a mouse which can easily cause wrist, elbow and shoulder problems. Our lives are more comfortable and we concentrate on mental development but lack balanced physical training. As a result, the upper body becomes very heavy and the lower body very weak. Even if a shop is just a few blocks away, most people will prefer to drive there. People will take the lift rather than take the stairs, even if only a few flights. In the airport, there are so many people who are sitting in a wheelchair instead of walking when they only have a small problem. Most people will stand on the moving sidewalk rather than walking along it to get to their gate faster.

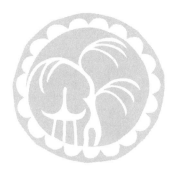

Because of this, more and more people have weaker legs and a heavy upper body, which will eventually cause problems in the joints. *Child Swinging* helps us to move our shoulders, elbows and wrists and helps us to develop the legs. This movement will also create strong circulation in the upper body and so it is very good for any injuries to the joints, like tennis elbow, frozen shoulder or stiffness in the neck.

HISTORY/BACKGROUND

Child Swinging actually comes from the Wing Chun movement, *Maan Sau*. Wing Chun is a martial art and so in the movement, *Maan Sau* we use more power and do not use the body to swing back and forth. *Child Swinging* is a Qigong movement and so we let the whole body connect with the movement. We also use the acupuncture points Quchi, which helps stimulate the large intestine channel and opens all the Qi in the arms and neck.

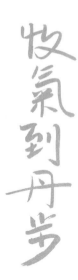

Collecting Qi to the Dantian – Walking

GOOD FOR • Coordination • Insomnia • Grounding the Qi

ACUPUNCTURE POINT Ren Channel (see page 64) and Laogong (see page 59)

1 Stand with your feet together and legs slightly bent. Place your hands at the Lower Dantian, the left hand over the right hand. Your back should be straight and arms loose.

2 Step to the right side with the right foot and at the same time move the right arm out to the side of the body. Your right palm faces forwards and your left arm should stay by your side.

3 Continue to move the right arm upwards to the Sky Eye (see page 66). As your right hand comes to the Sky Eye, start to shift the weight to the right side and lift up the left hand to the side of the body.

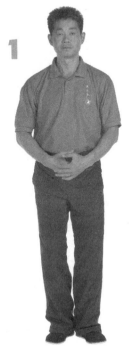

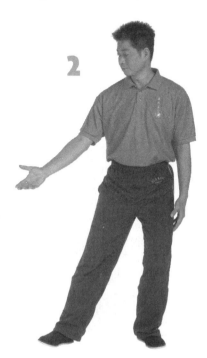

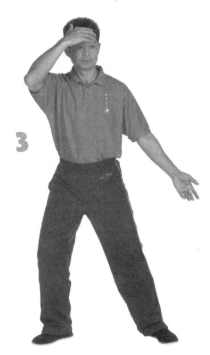

4 Simultaneously close your left foot next to the right foot and start to lower your right hand to the Lower Dantian and raise the left hand up to the Sky Eye.

5 Bring the left hand up to the Sky Eye and the right hand down to the Lower Dantian. Make sure to follow the Ren Channel as you lower the hand.

6 Repeat the same walking walking right foot/right hand, left foot/left hand for a total of six steps on each foot. Make sure that when one hand is at the Sky Eye, the other hand is at the Lower Dantian and feet are together. The hands should be balanced and move together. When you come to the last step, closing the left foot to the right foot, let both hands come back to the Dantian.

Exercise continues ➡

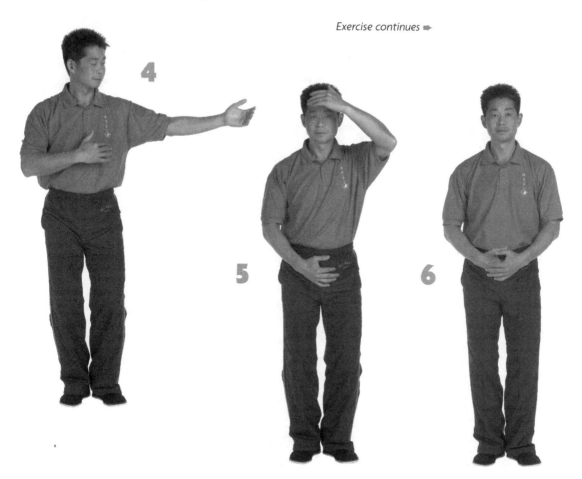

7 Start to walk back to the left, taking the same number of steps that you walked initially. You should first step with the left foot and lift up the left hand together.

8 Keep repeating the same exercise and walk back to the original starting place.

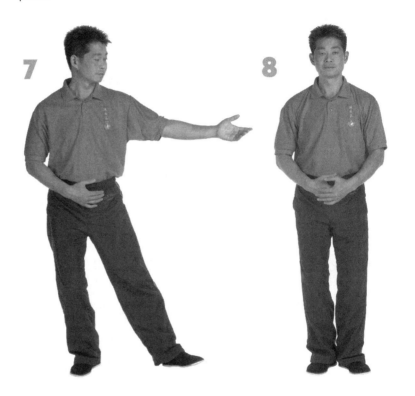

BREATHING

Throughout the whole movement, breathe naturally. You do not need to connect with the left hand to breathe in or right hand to breathe out as this is a sequence of movements.

CONCENTRATION

Make sure you move left hand and left leg together and right hand and right leg together. Throughout, make sure you keep your knees bent and the body at the same level. Do not move up and down as you step. Keep the eyes on the hand that is lifting.

BENEFITS

A lot of the time when we walk, we rush. If we walk too fast, we will use energy. In this exercise, you should walk slowly, so the Qi will go through all the channels slowly and cover every part of the body. That will help your mind and body to connect together because you are moving slowly.

As you bend your knees to walk, all your weight is on your thighs and your upper body will feel light. This will create a warm feeling in the body as the Qi is building up in the bones and marrow of the legs. Sometimes, however, your legs may be a little bit tired because you are keeping the knees bent the entire time, but this is a very good way to develop Qi and make the whole body strong and healthy.

At you move the arms, you are collecting energy. You should make sure that your palm faces and lowers down the Ren Channel (see page 64) and all the way down to the Lower Dantian. This way, every time you move, the energy will go down to the Lower Dantian and open the Ren Channel. This will benefit your circulation and help your liver because the liver is involved in blood circulation.

As you do the movement, make sure that you coordinate your hands and step.

HISTORY/BACKGROUND

This movement obviously comes from *Green Sea Swimming Dragon Gong* (a form in the Kunlun Dayan Qigong system), but the footwork is slightly different. When we do this movement, we keep collecting the Qi to the Lower Dantian with simple walking. In Healthy Living Gong, we have both stationary movements and walking movements, and these act like Yin and Yang to balance our Qi.

12

Meditation and Healing for the Body

EVERYTHING IN THE universe follows the law of movement and stillness. As human beings, we move and we also rest. Nature has its own times of movement and stillness, growing and resting. These are the seasons, like spring and winter. The Yin and Yang principle determines all.

In Qigong, movements such as we learned in Chapter 11 are followed by meditation so that we can store the Qi that we have gathered. Meditation is a state of consciousness, and unconsciousness, it is a way of relaxing, making the body quiet and letting everything go back to normal, without movement. The Chinese call meditation *Jing Gong*, which means Quiet Gong. It is good for gathering and settling down Qi and bringing Qi back to normal. That is the power of nature.

Qigong movement helps us open up the channels and acupuncture points, relax the muscles and loosen the joints and release negative energy. It is like shaking dust from our clothing, although the dust comes out of the body, not our clothing.

Meditation, however, allows the fresh Qi that we have gathered from our practise to settle down in the body and stay in our heart, lungs, kidneys and other internal organs. This is important, as the internal organs will then have a healthy supply of Qi that can be used when we are tired or ill. If we do not meditate after practising Qigong, the Qi we have gathered will not be stored. This would be like putting money into a pocket that has a hole in it.

If we practise meditation only, without doing movement first, it takes longer to stimulate the Qi in the body and to let any physical problems get better. Our joints and muscles will not be strong and we will not be able to rid our body of all the negative energy. Therefore, we should practise movement first before we do meditation. This is the best way.

When we are ill, if we only do meditation it will take much longer for the body to recover. This is because in the beginning, illness begins on an external level. You have a feeling that something is not quite right, like just before catching a cold or flu. Within a week, if we do not get rid of the sick Qi, it will go to our internal organs. If we still let the sick Qi stay there, it will eventually go to the bones and this is very difficult to get rid of.

When we move, negative energy can be released much quicker. I have a Qigong student who has suffered from the auto-immune disease lupus for the last seven years. He was doing fine until he stopped practising his Qigong, and then he had a relapse which affected his kidneys to such a point that he went into hospital in a critical condition for three weeks, having to have daily kidney dialysis. He said that he lost confidence and took bottles and bottles of every kind of medicine available, both conventional and alternative. He also tried different kinds of therapies and healings but none worked.

Michael Tse practising the Ma Bo (Horse Stance Meditation) in China.

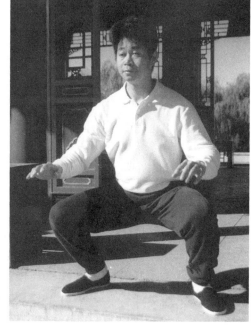

He contacted me to help him when I was doing a seminar near where he lived. After three treatments, he already felt his energy improve to a point where he could go back to his Qigong exercises and standing meditation (Ma Bo). He said that after building up to standing Qigong for twenty minutes a day, he had much more energy and was able to recover by himself. He asked me why the Qigong had not worked before and I explained to him that he had gone in too many directions, trying too many different things. Instead of trusting his Qigong, he tried too many different things. You need to trust and develop one thing to have success.

The standing meditation that he used is called Horse Stance and is an example of a Yang-style meditation. It is a meditation involving some movement, and because of this it is can be used as a Qigong movement as well as meditation. When I have any illness or injury, I do Horse Stance (Ma Bo) to help bring up the strong Qi to help the body to recover. I also get all of my patients and students to practise this method, as it will make the Qi very strong and make their other Qigong forms good.

In another case, one of my students had a shoulder problem and so I recommended he do the Healthy Living Gong movements *Separating the Fog to Look for the Clouds* and *Golden Dragon Stretches Its Claws* to help loosen the joints, and then to do sitting meditation. So every day, after his practice, he would do sitting meditation and found that it helped. This is a Yin type of meditation and can be used in combination with Yang type meditation practise.

Some people only practise meditation without doing any training of movement. Therefore, they are not strong, although their spirit may be high and the mind calmer. When these people only do meditation, they will have poor circulation and bad posture, particularly in the neck area. This is like having only one season, a winter without the summer. For the body to be balanced, you need both seasons.

Actually, we should cover both Yang and Yin, which is both movement and meditation. Movement is like hot summer and meditation is like a cool wind. This is a wonderful balance between Yin and Yang.

Ways of meditating

We have so many ways to practise meditation. We can do it lying down or sitting on a chair, stool or cushion. We can do standing or even lotus meditation. All of these different kinds of meditation, in the end, have the same benefit, although with some ways it may take longer to see the benefit.

Standing meditation is stronger than sitting meditation because when we stand, the Qi is very powerful and it makes the kidneys strong very quickly. Kidney energy is the first energy created from our Qigong practise. When the kidneys are healthy and strong, we will not feel tired. Our bones and teeth will be strong, our minds clear and our memory good.

Sitting meditation has a stronger effect than lying meditation. Sitting meditation is very good for helping the body to relax and heal injuries but should not replace standing meditation, as standing meditation will create very powerful Qi in the body. As for lying meditation, when you are lying down it takes much longer for the Qi to circulate in the body, and so usually I only recommend lying meditation as a beginning method for someone who is very ill and cannot stand. For healthy people, when you do lying meditation, you will often find that you fall asleep instead of doing meditation.

Lotus meditation is another method and it concentrates on bringing up the spiritual energy and circulating the Qi to benefit internal organs. Some people can sit for a long time in the lotus position if they have practised for a while. Some can even sit for several hours or even a day. However, for most people, this posture is unusual and is not so comfortable at first.

There are many different kinds of meditation in the style of Qigong which I teach. However, for the purposes of this book, I have tried to offer some simple methods which I think will benefit the most people, most of the time. Below are two different kinds of meditation. The first is a Yang meditation, called Ma Bo or Horse Stance. We do this one with the eyes open as it is a very powerful kind of meditation for both releasing the sick energy from the body and healing any problems. The second is a Yin, sitting meditation which is less strenuous but takes longer to heal the body.

The sitting meditation can be done on any straight-backed chair. The most important thing is to relax, keep the posture straight and breathe through the nose. This can be done anywhere and will make the mind calm and help heal any problems with the joints and back.

I always recommend Ma Bo to both my students and my patients. One of my patients who was diagnosed with kidney cancer came to me to ask if there was any Qigong method that he could use instead of having surgery or traditional treatment. He started with a few minutes of Ma Bo and built up to thirty minutes standing twice a day. This was over six years ago and he is still doing fine, without having had any cancer treatments.

I also do Ma Bo myself after I have treated patients, because when we do healing, we exchange Qi with that person. The more healthy you are and the more ill the patient, the more your good Qi will pass to them and the more sick Qi you will take on yourself. Unless you want this Qi to stay in your own body and cause problems, you need to release it. The quickest way I have found is to do Ma Bo. Because this particular Ma Bo posture is not just staying in one position, but moving up and down, it forces the Qi to became very powerful and clean up the body very, very quickly. Afterwards, you will feel good, just like when you were a child.

Ma Bo meditation

There are three positions for Ma Bo meditation: high, medium and low. In both the high and medium postures, the right posture is to keep the Baihui and Huiyin points in a straight line (see Chapter 9, 'Importance of Correct Posture'). In the low stance, the Baihui point and the Yongquan point should be in line. This is because when you are this low, it is not possible to keep the back in a straight line. However, in all of the postures, make sure that you keep your head up and eyes looking straight ahead.

1 Stand with the feet slightly wider than shoulder-width apart. Hold the arms to the side of the body. The forearms should be parallel to the ground and the palms facing the earth. Keep the mouth closed and tongue touching the upper palate. Eyes should look forward in a relaxed manner.

Keep the arms in the above position and bend the knees so that all the weight is on your thighs. Keep the back straight, so that the Baihui point and Huiyin points are in line. In the beginning, take a higher stance until your legs become stronger, then you can go lower.

2 When you feel comfortable, bend the knees a bit more so that you are in a medium Ma Bo stance.

3 If you want, you can even try to do a lower Ma Bo stance. Still keep the back straight and arms open and relaxed. Try to stay in this lower position for even a few seconds, then try to build up to a minute or longer if possible. When tired, gently go back to the higher position with knees still slightly bent. When we finish the exercise, we must wash the face Qigong style (see page 117) and then do what we call Shou Gong. This is for collecting all the Qi back to the Dantian to store in the body.

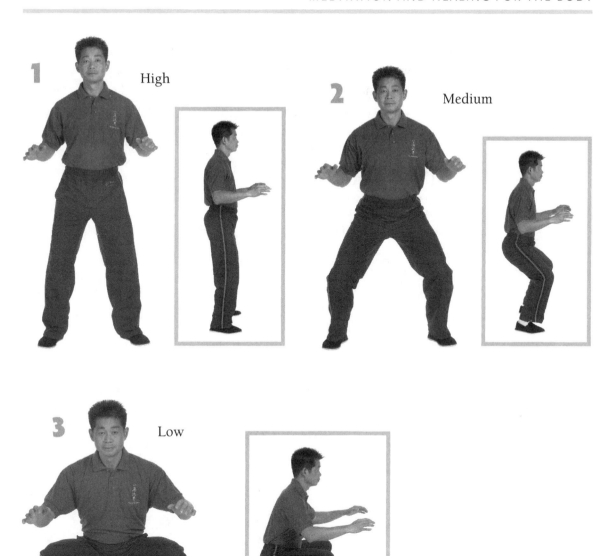

1 High

2 Medium

3 Low

Ma Bo is one of the treasures of Chinese skill and is a very powerful healing method. If you want to be very healthy and strong, do this every day and slowly increase the time that you practise it.

When doing Ma Bo, the most important thing is to keep your shoulders and arms relaxed and back straight. Do not tilt your hips forward as this will block the Qi and put the weight on the lower back instead of the legs. All the weight must be on the thighs for the Qi to develop properly. It will make your bones and kidneys stronger and will increase bone marrow. We keep the eyes open for this meditation because the Qi is very powerful. If you close the eyes, the body may start to move and you will lose Qi.

Sitting meditation

Sitting meditation is a Yin meditation and can be done anytime for relaxation and storing Qi after practising the Healthy Living Gong.

1 Sit forward on a straight-backed chair. Place both feet flat on the floor, shoulder-width apart. The toes should be in line with the front of the knees.

2 Place the palms on the thighs and relax the shoulders.

3 Close the mouth and close the eyes and try to empty the mind.

4 Relax the body from the top of the head, neck, shoulders, back, arms and

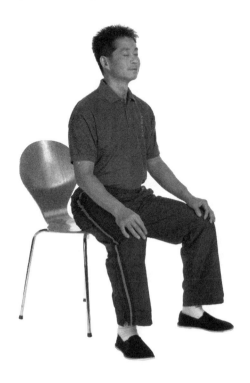

waist down to the toes. Keep the mouth closed and breathe through the nose. Try to empty the mind and just relax.

5 When finished, wash the face and do Shou Gong three times.

If you can meditate for five to 10 minutes, you will start to find a lot of benefit. In the future, you can even try to build up to 20 minutes. Meditating this long will help to heal all the illness and problems in the body, as well as store Qi.

Washing the face

1 Rub the palms of the hands together.

2 Brush the palms of the hands over the nose, eyes, top of head, ears and mouth three times.

When we do this, we are bringing Qi back to the five major internal organs through their external connections. The nose relates to the lungs, eyes to the liver, ears to the kidneys, mouth to the spleen and the tongue to the heart.

Exercise continues ➡

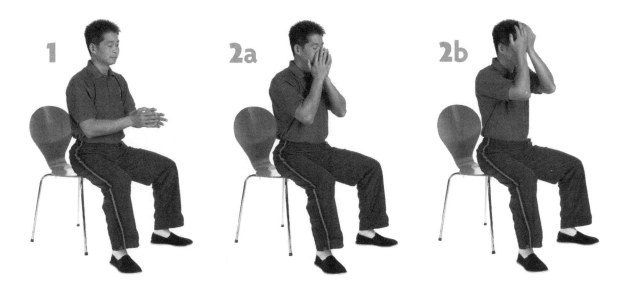

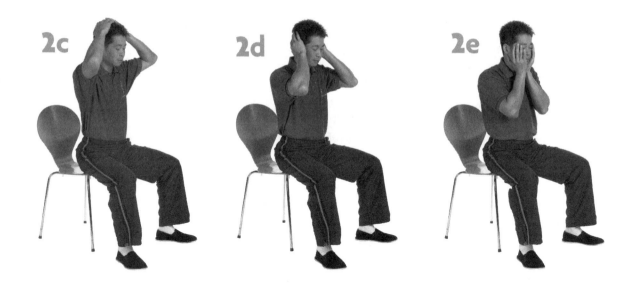

Shou Gong

Shou Gong is the movement we do when we have completely finished our Qigong exercises.

1 Stand with your feet shoulder-width apart.

2 Raise both hands to the side of the body up to shoulder height.

3 When your arms reach shoulder height, bend the elbows and bring the palms past the face, upper body and Dantian.

4 Lower hands down the Ren Channel and on to the Lower Dantian. Do this a further two times.

When you raise the arms, imagine you are gathering all the Qi from the heaven and pouring it into your body. Keep the Laogong points facing the body as you lower the hands past the face to the Lower Dantian. In this way, you open the Yang channels and then transmit Qi down the Yin channels of the body and back into the internal organs.

This is very good for relaxing the mind and body. We can also use this same movement at the beginning of our Qigong exercises, although when we do it in the beginning, we call it Relaxation Movement instead of Shou Gong.

If you can meditate for three to five minutes in the beginning, you are doing very well. You may find that your legs tremble. This is the body's way of releasing negative energy and opening the channels for stronger Qi. When you are tired, move to a higher stance and rest there for a while. Then go lower and stay for as long as you can before coming up again.

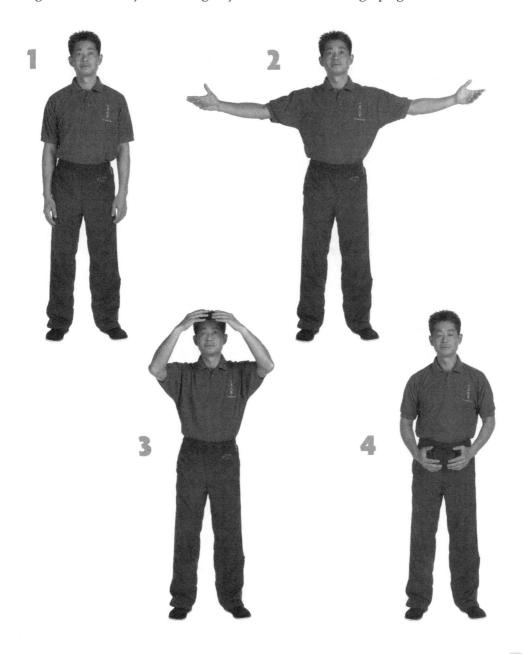

Glossary of Illnesses matched to Exercises

Health Problems	Exercise
Arthritis	Child Swinging,
	Golden Dragon Stretches Its Claws
Asthma	Holding the Beautiful Ball,
	Separating the Fog to Look for the Clouds
Backache	Looking for Treasure at the Bottom of the Chest
Breathing problems	Separating the Fog to Look for the Clouds
Bronchitis	Holding the Beautiful Ball,
	Separating the Fog to Look for the Clouds
Circulatory problems	Collecting Qi to the Dantian,
	Catching Fish by the Side of the Lake
Cold hands	Holding the Beautiful Ball
Coordination	Collecting Qi to the Dantian – Walking
	Golden Dragon Stretches Its Claws,
	Jade Ladder Climbing to the Sky
Dantian	Collecting Qi to the Dantian,
	Old Tree with Winding Roots
Depression	Separating the Fog to Look for the Clouds

Health Problems	Exercise
Digestion problems	Separating the Fog to Look for the Clouds
Finger injury	Golden Dragon Stretches Its Claws
Headache	Catching Fish by the Side of the Lake
Heart	Looking for Treasure at the Bottom of the Chest
High blood pressure	Jade Ladder Climbing to the Sky
Hips	Golden Dragon Stretches Its Claws
Insomnia	Collecting Qi to the Dantian
Kidneys weak	Looking for Treasure at the Bottom of the Chest Old Tree with Winding Roots
Knees	Child Swinging, Holding the Beautiful Ball, Golden Dragon Stretches Its Claws
Leg weakness	Old Tree with Winding Roots
Low blood pressure	Catching Fish by the Side of the Lake
Lungs	Separating the Fog to Look for the Clouds
ME (chronic fatigue syndrome)	Jade Ladder Climbing to the Sky
Memory problems	Collecting Qi to the Dantian, Meditation
Micro-cosmic orbit	Holding the Beautiful Ball
Posture	Jade Ladder Climbing to the Sky
Sexual dysfunction	Looking for Treasure at the Bottom of the Chest, Old Tree with Winding Roots
Shoulder problems	Child Swinging, Golden Dragon Stretches Its Claws
Stomach/spleen weakness	Separating the Fog to Look for the Clouds
Stress	Collecting Qi to the Dantian, Meditation
Tennis Elbow	Child Swinging

2 Letters from Practitioners of Healthy Living Gong

Over the last few years, I have heard from many people to say how practising Healthy Living Gong has helped them recover from some illness or generally improve their health and well being. Others have said that they are much more relaxed and can concentrate better at work and sleep better at night. Below are a few of the letters that I have received from students and which I hope will encourage you in your own practising.

Multiple sclerosis

About 15 years ago, Western doctors diagnosed me with multiple sclerosis, supposedly a debilitating neurological disease which progresses until one loses control of many physical functions. In the first 10 years, I did experience problems with ambulation, vision, numbness and tingling, weakness of the arms and legs, and indeed needed to be hospitalised twice and treated as an outpatient several times with massive doses of steroids.

I began to study Qigong six years ago but it was only two years ago that I finally decided to wholly commit myself to practising Qigong. I can only now appreciate, as I reflect on how Healthy Living Gong (HLG) has impacted on my life, how critical it was in helping me to balance and relax. It feels so good to do *Old Tree with Winding Roots*.

When my Sifu, Adam Wallace, began teaching HLG, I was puzzled by why we were learning what seemed to me at first to be simpler, more fundamental exercises than the more challenging *Wild Goose* forms which I had already learned. It became clear by the time I had begun to learn the movement *Jade Ladder Climbing to the Sky* that this family of exercises was very important and powerful. It was certainly subtle and now I realise quite amazingly how much HLG helps with everyday activities as well as when practising more complex Qigong forms.

Several years ago my neurologist reviewed the results of an MRI brain scan with me, and it revealed that one very large lesion had virtually disappeared. He did not have a medical explanation, but just commented that such changes can occur. That night at class, with MRI films in hand, I ran into class and hugged Sifu and thanked him for helping me to stay healthy. It was a wonderful moment! I also treasure a moment I had during my last visit to the neuro-ophthalmologist. He has always been impressed with how active my lifestyle is and happy that my vision has been fairly stable, yet he still encourages me to consider taking medication. I told him, 'no', once again and urged him to write one simple word in my chart... '*Qigong*'.

MAUREEN MADDEN
Student, New York

Insomnia and over-thinking

How does one describe Healthy Living Gong and how do I distinguish it from the other Qigong exercises I have learned like *Balancing Gong*, *Green Sea Swimming Dragon Gong*, *Jade Pillar Gong* or any of the other forms within the Kunlun Dayan system? Language fails to accurately describe subjective experience. Only by personal contact can one begin to understand the nature of something simple yet complex.

After consistent practice and the development of a relaxed awareness during the Healthy Living Gong exercises, one begins to feel the difference of each of the movements. Although similar (all fingerprints look the same upon superficial examination), each movement has a unique 'stamp' that gives it a particular feeling, flavour and purpose.

For me, the special character of Healthy Living Gong is *calmness* and *relaxation*. When I practise, I feel all the tension release from my body. I feel rooted to the earth and a part of nature, not an unrelated fragment spinning out of control! For me, Healthy Living Gong is like a moving meditation, so I often use it to centre myself. Life is too fast – brimming with responsibilities, multi-tasking, and over-thinking, especially with three children and a full-time job. So it is wonderful to be able to return to a place of stillness, to gather energy from nature, to remember we are a part of something real.

Besides being good for relaxation, it is also helpful for quelling a variety of unpleasant physical symptoms. I have used it many times after waking in the middle of the night with insomnia or digestive problems (acid reflux). The exercise *Collecting Qi to the Dantian* is excellent for moving Qi from wherever it is causing a disturbance back to where it belongs (the Lower Dantian). It is amazing, but after about fifteen minutes of practise, any discomfort is resolved. Since practising Qigong, I don't feel as anxious or upset about physical disturbances any more, because I know that I have a tool that I can use to help myself.

Each of the exercises in the set has a specific purpose. Among these are exercises that gently stretch the body (improving flexibility), improve balance and posture, and stimulate the internal organs and acupuncture points. This helps enable Qi to flow unimpeded over time, helping to clear blockages and improve health. The exercises also release endorphins which leave one with a feeling of calm and well-being.

ADAH MASAOKA
Student, Seattle

Golfer with tennis elbow and high blood pressure

I have attended the Manchester classes for about 18 months now. The longer I spend there, the more I feel I ought to write down the benefits I have enjoyed from studying Qigong. After having by-pass surgery, Qigong has proven to be the most suitable exercise for me I have ever seen.

My regular check-ups, including my blood pressure, have shown that Qigong has really helped. I have a sense of growing confidence and well-being which I have not experienced before. Aches and pains which I took for granted have disappeared, although once in a while they reappear after a particularly hard workout for a short while.

I also play golf in my spare time and my ability to perform well at it has not decreased with age. I'm convinced that Qigong has made a big contribution here. I was surprised when over a period of time of about one month, my golfer's or tennis elbow disappeared completely during the time I was studying Healthy Living Gong. One of the instructors (Simon) explained that the movement *Child Swinging* was a treatment for tennis elbow and for repetitive strain injury. I have had no trouble from it ever since.

I am writing this letter partly because I hope it will give encouragement to anyone just beginning to study Qigong. As long as the student persists and practises, then he or she can enjoy its many therapeutic benefits. Finally, I would like to thank all the instructors and students at the Tse Qigong Centre for their help and friendliness.

Yours sincerely,
DAVID FAWKES
Student, Manchester

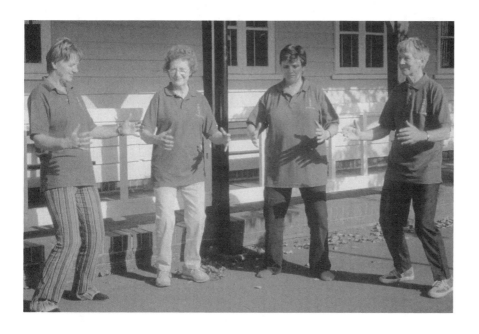

Knee and back injury recovery

I began studying Qigong just over a year ago. My close friend Derek had the honour of learning directly under Sigong (Grandteacher) Michael Tse while he was living in the Seattle area. Over time I began to notice some definite changes in my friend. He had always been in good physical shape, but I'd noticed that his fiery spirit had begun to noticeably calm down and that he seemed to be making a more deliberate effort to better himself as a person.

This was very interesting to me. Myself, I always had respect for Kung Fu and thought perhaps that one day when the time was right I would begin training. The years had taken a toll on my young body, though. I have been a landscaper for 10 years and previous to that I had played American football for six years and generally worked my body very hard with basketball and hiking and other athletic endeavours. I was also struggling with two health problems. The first was a badly hyper-extended knee.

I'd hurt it the previous winter going snowboarding for my first time. It now had a terrible habit of popping out of joint when I'd flex it too far, and it was healing very slowly. The other problem was a bit more serious. I've had back problems ever since I was 17 years old, and on occasion I would be completely laid out and unable to work for up to a week or so. After the worst bout with my back I'd ever had (where I was unable to work for three months while trying various suggestions to get it healthy again), I finally succumbed and went to a back specialist.

He looked at my X-rays and told me that the previous diagnoses had been wrong, and that I had degenerative disc disease at the age of 25. He said it was fairly common in America but that it had no cure. My case was apparently a minor one, but he went on to explain that it usually gets worse over time and sometimes quite quickly. The doctors had been telling me to rest my back before, but he told me that I needed to exercise regularly, and that I should avoid any high impact sports (such as basketball or difficult hikes). He also told me that I should consider a new line of work. That was all he 'knew' about it though.

I was sceptical, to say the least, at this so-called 'expert' telling me that I had an incurable disease that they knew little or nothing about, that I needed to change my entire lifestyle and accept that I probably would not have my previous health back ever again.

I wasn't ready to give up my athletics, so I determined it was time for a different approach. I had spoken with Derek a few times about his Qigong and I decided to go ahead and give it a try. Soon afterwards, I started my first class at the Seattle Tse Qigong Centre under Sifu Adah Masaoka. In the beginning, I was nervous. When I was younger I had sat in on a Karate class and a Tae Kwon Do class to see what they were like. I had been turned off by the competitive nature between the students and the 'drill-sergeant' styles of the instructors. They really distanced themselves from the students and seemed to almost look down on them as their inferiors.

I quickly found that this was not at all the case in this class. The students were all very calm and even-tempered. They were polite and friendly and more than willing to take the time to help me out with things. Sifu Adah Masaoka moved me along at a comfortable speed and treated me with respect. She taught without the arrogance that teachers sometimes fall prey to. She was humble before the skill and I couldn't help but to be humble before her example. I felt right at home and quickly decided to carry on with the Qigong to see for myself how it would affect me.

A few months later I had passed my test for Balancing Gong and started Healthy Living Gong. My knee had already shown a marked improvement in flexibility, although it would still pop out of joint if I stretched it too far. My back was still sore at times, but I hadn't had to miss any work since I had started the Qigong, and it seemed to be growing stronger, although I wasn't ready to test it out fully yet. Healthy Living Gong quickly proved to be a bit more challenging than Balancing Gong had been.

The movements were slightly more complex and required more subtle control and finesse. More balance and flexibility was required for most of the movements. Also, more strength was required. Each step seemed to prepare me for the next step though. Almost immediately my knees seemed to be growing stronger and stronger. Before too long, my back wasn't giving me any trouble at all unless I sat with bad posture for a long time or slept in a funny position.

I also began to grow much more aware of my body and started to realise how much tension I was carrying (especially in my lower back, shoulders and neck), even when I thought I was just relaxing. However, this also began to improve slowly. By the time I had started on more advanced Healthy Living Gong my knee was up to about 90 per cent. It had no more pain, and nearly the same mobility it had before the injury. It still would sometimes make a deep 'pop' if I flexed it all the way and held it that way for too long, but it wasn't affecting my lifestyle any more.

My Qigong seemed to have helped my basketball, as well, making me more aware of how my body moved and thereby giving me better control over it. The Qigong seeds are planted inside me now, and I have no doubt that they will one day grow into something special. With more diligent practise and a few other steps towards living healthier, I am sure that both the quality and the length of my life will only increase. That is a priceless gift and one that I am very thankful for. I am still but a novice and have yet to feel the full potential of these skills, but I've had a taste of them and I've learned to recognise the skill in those above me. If there is a ceiling to Qigong skill, it is high up in the clouds and far beyond the range of these eyes. Still, I am amazed that with as little as a month of dedicated practice, you can still get definite benefits. You can climb the Qigong tree as high as you want to go, but the view only keeps getting better with every step!

GABRIEL McCALLUM
Student, Seattle

Kidney failure and coma

Right now I am sitting here writing this letter by a gorgeous lake in New York State. Two years ago, I never thought that I would be here again. As a matter of fact, I am lucky to be alive right now. Several years ago, I developed an illness that affected my kidneys. I first used conventional medicine but it did not offer any cure. So I then tried holistic medicine. I must have spent over $50,000 in the last few years trying to find the best healer in the world who could help me. I listened to anybody and everybody who said that they would cure me. Eventually, I wound up in worse shape than I began. I ended up in hospital, in a coma and on dialysis. I also went into kidney failure.

I never realised how weak a person's body could be. After three weeks, I awoke from the coma and the doctors discharged me from the hospital. I had to walk with a cane and could barely walk several feet without assistance. This was December of 2001. In March of 2002, Sifu Michael Tse came to my area in New York City. Although I was too weak to attend his seminar, I saw him for three Qigong healing treatments. I could not believe the difference in how I felt afterwards. It was a miracle and the best that I had felt in years.

Tse Sifu cautioned me that the energy that he transmitted to me was only a 'jump start' and that I had to keep on practising my exercises to maintain my level of health. So, he instructed me to do the Horse Stance meditation. He said to do as long as I could, even if only a minute or two and then gradually build up to 30 minutes, and to start doing some of the basic Qigong exercises that I had learned several years before.

Within several weeks of my treatments, Qigong practise and doing the Horse Stance, I was off dialysis and back to work as a police officer. The doctors were amazed at my progress.

I truly believe that Qigong has helped me tremendously. I also learned recently that Qigong is not to be done like most exercises, like lifting weights or doing aerobics where you perform repetitions quite robotically. Adam Wallace, a Centre instructor here in New York, has taught me that the most important thing to do is to relax and to breathe naturally.

I once read that Sifu said that it is better to have one sharp knife than a drawer full of dull knives. I truly believe this. Before, I used too many approaches to maintain my health instead of sticking to just one that really helped me the most – the exercises which are part of the Kunlun Dayan Qigong system.

With highest regards,
Jim Collis
Student, New York

Index

To contact Michael Tse:

UK
Tse Qigong Centre
PO Box 59
Altrincham WA15 8FS
Tel. 0161 929 4485
Email: tse@qimagazine.com
www.qimagazine.com

USA
Tse Qigong Centre
PO Box 15807
Honolulu, HI 96830
Tel. 808 528 8501
Email: tse@wildgooseqigong.com
www.qimagazine.com